INTERMITTENT FASTING DIET
GUIDE + COOKBOOK

Dr. Becky Gillaspy

Recipes by Lovoni Walker

ALPHA

Penguin
Random
House

Publisher Mike Sanders
Editor Alexandra Andrzejewski
Designer and Art Director Rebecca Batchelor
Photographer and Food Stylist Lovoni Walker
Recipe Developer Lovoni Walker
Recipe Tester Irena Shnayder
Proofreaders Christy Wagner, Georgette Beatty
Indexer Brad Herriman

First American Edition, 2020
Published in the United States by DK Publishing
6081 E. 82nd Street, Indianapolis, IN 46250

ISBN: 978-1-4654-9766-6

Library of Congress Catalog Number: 2020931125

DK books are available at special discounts when purchased
in bulk for sales promotions, premiums, fund-raising,
or educational use. For details, contact:
SpecialSales@dk.com

Printed and bound in Canada

Photograph on page 224 © Steve Miller Photography
All other images © Dorling Kindersley Limited

For the curious

www.dk.com

To Keith, I've been blessed to walk through life with you.

CONTENTS

What if I told you about an investment you could make in your health that required you to do less rather than more? What if this investment did not cost a dime, but instead likely saved you money? Imagine a weight-loss strategy that folded into your normal routine and allowed you to eat with family and friends, even if they weren't following your "diet." Picture making no changes to your food choices or exercise routine, yet stepping on the scale to find you've lost weight. Not only has the scale moved, but you have also realized that you are sleeping more soundly and have more energy.

INTRODUCTION

It sounds far-fetched, but these are the results that a group of research study participants got when they did nothing more than shorten the number of hours per day during which they consumed food.[1] The same benefits await you when you practice intermittent fasting (IF).

What Is Intermittent Fasting?

Intermittent fasting is not so much a diet as it is a timing strategy. In its most basic form, IF requires you to do nothing more than split your day between a period of eating and not eating (fasting). If you can stop eating a few hours before bed and push breakfast back a few hours, you can do intermittent fasting.

Why Does It Work?

It sounds too simple to be effective, but intermittent fasting works because drawing a clear line between eating and fasting allows you to work with your body's natural metabolic rhythm. When you're intermittently fasting and your eating window is open, you will be consuming calories (a.k.a. energy) at a time when your body is best equipped to handle them. The human body is designed to be active during daylight hours and to sleep at night. We refer to this daily cycle as your *circadian rhythm*—the internal clock that helps you keep this wake/sleep cycle on track, which is found in your brain and takes its cue from light. However, there are also accessory clocks found in your organs, and they take their cues from your food intake. When you start eating, you wake up these digestive clocks and they go to work, helping you digest, absorb, release, and store energy efficiently. However, the clocks in these metabolically important organs wind down as your day progresses.

The result is that the foods you eat at the beginning of your eating day are handled more efficiently than those consumed later in the day. By shortening the number of hours during which you consume food, you work with your body's natural rhythm and become a more efficient metabolic machine. During your fasting period, you'll be giving your digestive system a rest, which resets the hormones that impact your weight. This rest period also frees up resources that your body can use for cleanup and repair.

It all comes back to hormones, the mail carriers of your body—the messages they carry tell your cells what to do. When your body is busy digesting food, hormones are produced to help you use the energy from that food. If you consume more energy than you need at the moment, hormones play a role in storing the excess for later in places such as adipose (fat) tissue. That's how body fat grows.

However, when you fast, those fat-storing hormones quiet down, allowing fat to be released from your fat cells, which is how body fat shrinks. When you have food in your stomach, many resources get diverted to the digestive tract to deal with the nutrients—digestion is an energy-demanding process. When you fast, those resources are freed up, allowing important repair processes to take place that lower your risk of certain diseases, boost your brain function, delay aging, and, yes, also help you lose weight.[2]

Your body's natural clocks

The master clock in your brain wakes you up with the morning light and makes you sleepy at night.

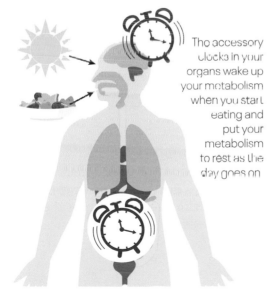

The accessory clocks in your organs wake up your metabolism when you start eating and put your metabolism to rest as the day goes on

When you practice intermittent fasting, you consume calories during the hours of the day that your body is best able to handle them.

I'll Be Your Fasting Coach

With this book, you'll learn why intermittent fasting works for weight loss and better health and how you can fit fasting into your life. I'll be your coach through this process. I will show you what to do to maximize your results. Together, we will challenge some well-established beliefs (like is breakfast really the most important meal of the day?) and uncover shortcuts to better health and the enjoyment of life. You'll discover for yourself that intermittent fasting has a "stickiness" factor, meaning that those who give it a try tend to stick with it because the effort is small, but the rewards are great.

This book is action ready. I don't just explain why IF is an easy, enjoyable, and effective path to better health and weight loss; I also set you up with recipes and meal plans to eliminate all of the guesswork. You'll receive a complete "I can do this" strategy.

In Part 1, you'll learn the ins and outs of intermittent fasting. You'll discover what happens inside your body when you fast and be given glimpses into how fasting feels as I share insights from those already doing it. You'll be introduced to different fasting strategies, and I'll guide you through selecting the one that will benefit you most. Part 2 of the book is when you get to put your knowledge into action. You'll be given meal plans and recipes that clearly show you what to eat and drink during your eating hours. In other words, the hard work of planning is done for you!

I'm excited to share the art and science of IF with you and can't wait for you to experience the health and weight loss rewards that come from this easy-to-follow strategy. Turn the page, and let's take the first step together.

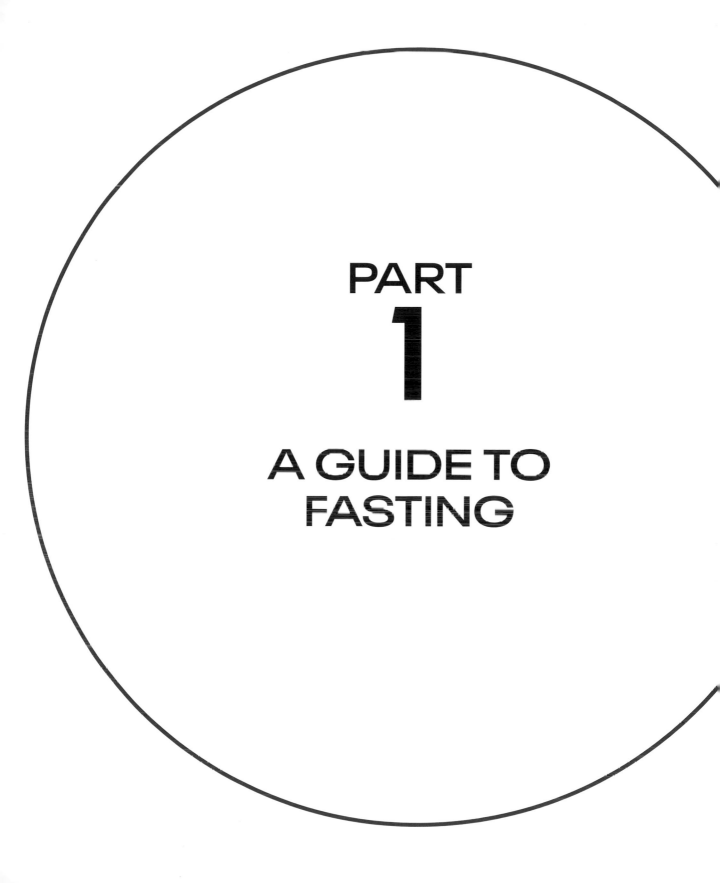

PART
1

A GUIDE TO
FASTING

1

THIS IS HOW WE EAT

What lies ahead

- **How we think we eat does not match how we actually eat.** Most people are really eating from the moment they wake up until the moment their head hits the pillow at night that's more than 15 hours for some! Moreover, we typically eat far more calories than we would have guessed.

- **You might want to move away from the several-small-meals-a-day routine.** Frequent eating puts our metabolic processes into overdrive, not giving our bodies time to rest.

- **Is it safe to skip breakfast?** Most people can successfully skip breakfast without the risk of gaining weight or slowing their metabolism.

Do you wake up with the best intentions of healthfulness, eating a bowl of oatmeal and an apple with your morning coffee? But then do you go to bed just after finishing off a third glass of wine and a few innocent squares of chocolate? Challenging these long-ingrained habits could be just the key to healing your metabolism and helping you to shed pounds.

MISREPORTING WHAT WE EAT

We are notoriously bad at estimating our food intake. To detect just how bad we are at this seemingly simple skill, researchers treated a group of adults to an all-American fast-food meal consisting of a hamburger, fries, and ice cream. After the meal, participants were asked to estimate how much they ate. How did they do? Not so well. They underreported the portion size of every food they ate, and they underestimated their calorie intake by up to 40 percent.[1]

We also don't like revealing the times we indulge in less-than-wholesome foods, such as sweet treats and buttery biscuits. Yet we have no problem sharing our healthy habits. "Cookies? Oh, I eat them occasionally, but kale is what I really love!" So, whether we are reluctant to report foods we think are unhealthy, or whether we innocently misremember our food choices, when asked to recall our recent food intake, few of us earn high marks for accuracy.[2]

These tendencies to underreport what and how often we eat create problems for nutrition researchers, who often lament "How do we scientifically evaluate whether your four-soda-a-day habit is impacting your health if you don't tell us you drink them?" Yet, with no better option available, researchers have continued to plug away for decades, relying on food frequency and diet history questionnaires that ask people to recall things like:

Over the past 12 months, how often did you drink milk as a beverage (NOT in coffee, tea, or cereal; including soy, rice, almond, and coconut milk; NOT including chocolate milk, hot chocolate, and milkshakes)?

- *1 time per month or less*
- *2–3 times per month*
- *1–2 times per week*
- *3–4 times per week*
- *5–6 times per week*
- *1 time per day*
- *2–3 times per day*
- *4–5 times per day*
- *6 or more times per day*[3]

Ummm?

To make matters worse, once you get through that question, you are faced with 140 more pages of questions. Is anyone else feeling sleepy right now?

Enter the age of the smartphone. Thanks to the advent of technology, a better way to evaluate the eating habits of the public is within grasp. Dr. Satchin Panda is a researcher who has studied the relationship between our food intake and our natural circadian rhythm, which is that internal clock inside our head that tells us when to sleep and when to be active. Much of the research he has performed has been on mice. The diet of a mouse is easy to study because we control what and how much it eats. But there are stark differences between how mice and humans live their lives. At some point, we must take what we've learned from mice and try it out on humans.

Knowing the shortfalls of food questionnaires, Dr. Panda came up with an innovative app that allows people to report their food intake using the camera on their smartphone. Although it could still be hard to bring yourself to snap a picture of the empty chip bag you just devoured, the research team found that this method improves reporting accuracy, providing a much clearer picture of how you eat. As it turns out, more than half of us are all-day grazers, eating for 15 hours or longer every day and taking a break only to catch some shut-eye. We also eat the majority of our calories (more than 35%) at night after 6pm. When it comes to the weekend, we eat differently than we do on weekdays, creating what the research team termed "metabolic jetlag" that is similar to the jetlag we experience when flying across time zones.[4]

SHIFTING OUR EATING WINDOW

This glimpse into our eating habits is interesting by itself, but what's truly eye-opening is what happened when a group of the study's participants reduced their eating duration by just a few hours.

Eight overweight individuals were recruited to take part in a 16-week intervention study. They were asked to reduce their eating duration for the day—which had been greater than 14 hours—down to 10 to 12 hours of their choosing. The participants were not given deliberate instructions or restrictions concerning their food choices or calorie intake; they were simply asked to consume all of their daily calories within a shortened time frame. By the end of the intervention, the participants had lost an average of 7.2 pounds (3.27kg) and reported their sleep satisfaction and energy levels had substantially improved. The changes these participants experienced were so impactful that they all voluntarily opted to continue unsupervised for an additional 36 weeks

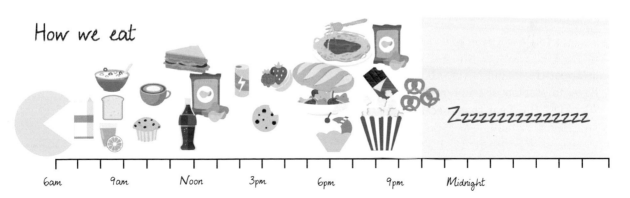

How we eat

6am   9am   Noon   3pm   6pm   9pm   Midnight

Most of us are all-day grazers. More than 50 percent of us eat for 15 hours or longer a day, stopping only to sleep. We also eat late at night, consuming most of our daily calories (more than 35%) after 6pm.

to complete a full year of eating within a shortened eating window. After 1 year, despite making no other (reported) changes to their eating habits, the participants maintained their weight loss, sleep, and energy benefits.[4]

If we are asked to describe our eating habits, many of us will proclaim that we eat three meals a day with an occasional snack thrown in here and there. This study revealed a different picture. In reality, many of us graze and grab food and drink, from the time we get up to the time we go to bed. This mindless eating pattern plays a role in the growing obesity epidemic that we face as a society, but this study also hints at a solution. By simply paying attention to when you start and stop eating, you can positively impact your weight and health. In other words, by consciously reducing the number of hours throughout the day that you eat, you unconsciously lose weight and improve your health.

THE THREE-MEAL-A-DAY CULTURE

When I was in ninth grade, I had an embarrassing problem. That year, I was assigned to the latest lunch period. I would eat breakfast before the school bus picked me up at 7am and then have to wait until almost 1pm to eat lunch. I felt like I was starving on a daily basis, and my stomach wanted to prove to everyone in my pre-lunchtime class that I was, in fact, on the verge of starvation by growling loudly for all ears to hear. As a shy girl who took comfort in not making a scene, these daily gurgles and groans brought giggles and sideways looks that made me want to cringe. My solution was to eat *more!* I theorized that the more food I could force into my stomach before the school bus came, the longer I could go without the growls. Breakfast went from being an enjoyable few minutes of downtime before the start of my busy day to being a laser-focused attempt to shove as many bowls of cereal into my body as humanly possible. However, despite my heroic attempts, no amount of cereal seemed to do the trick, and I trudged noisily through the remaining months of the semester. (By the way, I now know that the low-fiber, refined cereals that I loved as a kid take very little to digest. So, even though I ate a lot, the quick-digesting food left my system fast.)

I was in high school in the 1980s. I look at the '80s as a transition decade, and no, I am not referring to the transition to big hair and disco music, both of which I took part in. What I am referring to is a transition in the way we viewed food. During this decade, we saw a rising number of women joining the workforce and a new awareness about nutrition. With both parents working outside the home, a need arose for convenient, less time-consuming ways to feed the family. The first Dietary Guidelines for Americans was published in 1980 as a way to help American families make healthy food and beverage choices. This heightened public focus on nutrition led to some catchphrases and mantras that persist to this day, including "breakfast is the most important meal of the day."

With my failed attempts at eating a big enough breakfast to control "hunger," it seemed utterly ridiculous for me to consider skipping breakfast. If anything, I thought I needed two breakfasts rather than one!

Fast fact: why does my stomach growl?

A growling stomach is not necessarily a sign of hunger. Hunger is a hormonally driven communication between your gut and your brain. The gurgles and sounds you hear coming from inside you are most likely related to the digestion of food that goes on for hours after you eat.

Your digestive tract is lined with smooth muscles. When you eat something, these muscles contract to mix the food with digestive juices so you can get the nutrients out of the food. This movement is a noisy process, but when there is food in your system, the sound is muffled. During fasting, the muscles of the stomach and the small intestine are largely inactive. However, the muscles experience cycles of contractions that play a housekeeping role to clean out residual contents like mucus, food particles, and bacteria so your system is prepared for its next meal. These stomach contractions make noise. With no food in your system, your hollow digestive tract acts as an echo chamber, and you hear all of the gurgles and groans and growls that you associate with hunger.[5]

So I joined the chorus of breakfast supporters singing the well-known lyrics, including "breakfast jump-starts your metabolism" and "if you skip it, you'll overeat later in the day." Those beliefs were so ingrained in my mind that I never stopped to consider if they were facts or myths.

We live in a world of sound bites where much of our nutritional advice comes in 30-second commercials and 5-minute segments on morning talk shows. We tend to hear the same things so often that we adopt them as facts. As I learned and we will explore together, finding your path to better health and weight control requires some paradigm-shifting in regard to how we've been taught to eat. Let's start by looking at breakfast.

BREAKFAST: WHAT IF WE SKIP IT?

The greatest praise that I hear about eating breakfast is that it stimulates your metabolism and gets you ready for your day. Eating indeed gives you a metabolic boost, so there is something to that statement. However, the "boost" is more like a little bump—breakfast is not the metabolic jump-start that it is credited to be. When you eat food, whether it is in the form of breakfast, lunch, dinner, or a muffin from the snack cart, your digestive system springs into action to break down the food and distribute the nutrients. This process requires a lot of energy and as a result produces heat. That heat-producing reaction is known as the *thermic effect of food,* and it raises your metabolism above your normal level. However, the degree to which this raises your metabolism is small, so we can't say that eating breakfast is the definitive factor that revs up your metabolism and primes you for the day ahead. The credit for that feat goes to a complex interaction between your nervous system and hormones.

A few hours before you open your eyes in the morning, your body is busily preparing for the new day. This process of waking up is orchestrated by a complex ensemble of events that causes your body temperature and blood pressure to rise. As the day nears dawn, your body releases a host of wake-up hormones, including cortisol, which helps regulate your metabolism and aids you in responding to stress.[6, 7]

Even if we acknowledge that breakfast is not the metabolic gas pedal of our day, we have to consider what skipping it does to the rest of our day. A common notion is that skipping breakfast causes a rebound effect that makes you overeat later in the day. It seems logical that skipping breakfast will increase your hunger at lunchtime. It is also logical to assume that the hungrier you are, the more calories you'll consume.

There is research that supports the assertion that we eat more at lunch when we skip breakfast.[8] However, the extra lunchtime calories might not be enough to match the calories you missed out on by skipping breakfast. To test this theory, researchers recruited individuals to participate in a study. The participants were split into two groups, with one group asked to skip breakfast and the other served a large breakfast and allowed to eat as much as they wanted. The breakfast eaters consumed an average of 624 calories in the morning. When the two groups were invited to lunch that same day, the breakfast skippers rated their hunger significantly higher than the breakfast eaters—no surprise there. The skippers also ate more than those who had breakfast, but only 174 calories more. At the end of the day, those who skipped breakfast had a net calorie deficit of 450 calories.[9] This study and others like it do not support the notion that skipping breakfast contributes to a higher total calorie count for the day or weight gain.[10]

Fast fact: cortisol

You may have heard of cortisol described as "the stress hormone" that is released when you are under stress and that contributes to belly fat. This can lead you to believe that you always want levels of cortisol to be low. However, cortisol has important functions. For one thing, it helps you wake up in the morning. So, when your body is working properly, you'll see that cortisol peaks in the morning and then steadily declines over the course of the day, reaching its lowest point at bedtime, which allows you to get a good night's rest.

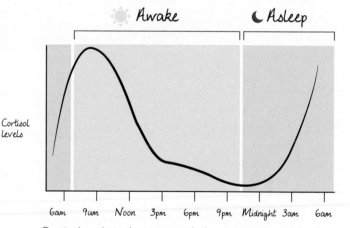

Cortisol peaks in the morning, helping you wake up and face the activities of your day. After the peak, cortisol steadily declines, reaching its low point at night, helping you sleep, before beginning to rise again for the next morning.

Quite the contrary, we see that skipping breakfast might reduce our overall daily calorie intake.

Many of the reasons we have for eating breakfast are not rooted in science, but rather mantras we've heard so often we've adopted them as fact. Indeed, it is not necessary for everyone to eat breakfast, but that doesn't mean everyone *should* ditch breakfast. Moreover, you don't need to be a breakfast skipper to practice intermittent fasting.

WHO SHOULD EAT BREAKFAST?

If you are taking a medication that requires eating food in the morning, then breakfast is the right choice for you. You might also find that you don't feel well or experience low blood sugar, shakiness, or fatigue when you skip breakfast, making the practice unwise. Breakfast is best thought of as "break fast," and you can do that at any hour of the day. As you start to put intermittent fasting into practice, you will find that it is a flexible strategy. So, whether you decide to skip breakfast or shorten your eating duration in other ways, you can benefit from fasting.

Is it okay to skip breakfast?

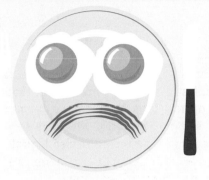

* **I thought breakfast jump-started my metabolism?** You get a small metabolic boost from eating, but hormones are what wake you up and prepare you for your day.

* **Will skipping breakfast cause me to overeat later in the day?** Studies show breakfast skippers might eat more at lunch, but their overall daily calorie intake is lower compared to breakfast eaters.

* **Is skipping breakfast okay for everyone?** No. If you feel unwell without breakfast or you take a medication with food, you should eat breakfast. Children might benefit mentally and physically when they eat breakfast.

* **Will I lose muscle if I skip breakfast?** The short fast that occurs when you skip a meal does not result in a loss of muscle protein. More on this in Chapter 3.

2

WHY FAST + WHO SHOULD DO IT?

What lies ahead

- **Intermittent fasting has a "stickiness" factor.** It is realistic to adhere to because of the three E's—easy to do, enjoyable, and effectivo.

- **Fasting "hacks" your biology.** You can influence how your body uses energy from food to influence weight loss, health, and well-being.

- **It's a good strategy for most people, but others must use caution.** Those with a history of eating disorders or other special concerns should be careful.

It's no question that diets can be difficult. Even pure, brute willpower is often not enough to tip the scale. If you're looking for the ever-elusive solution to your weight-loss woes, intermittent fasting may be the most practical, flexible, and effective strategy you have ever tried. It's not perfect for everyone, but read through the chapter to learn if it's right for you.

WHY WE STICK WITH FASTING

I like to say that intermittent fasting has a "stickiness" factor. What I mean by that is that once people give it a try, they tend to stick with it. That alone separates IF from other weight-loss and health strategies. Who among us can raise their hand and say they've never faltered on a diet or lost weight only to gain it back again because they couldn't stomach another rice cake or bland piece of boneless, skinless chicken breast? Many of us have joined gyms and never worked out or bought treadmills that turned into very expensive clothing racks.

Intermittent fasting is different. It folds easily into your daily life even when you're on vacation or celebrating the holidays. Although fasting works best when you pair it with a high-quality diet, this timing technique allows for a little wiggle room. Are you heading into the holidays and craving a piece of Grandma's pumpkin pie? You can work an intermittent fasting strategy around a holiday meal that will prevent you from losing too much ground. Are you tired of gaining weight when you go on vacation? In Chapter 7, I'll share an intermittent fasting strategy that I use when I travel to prevent weight gain. Have you tried complicated diet plans that required you to buy expensive ingredients only to be left feeling hungry and poor? If so, intermittent fasting will feel like a breath of fresh air. If conventional strategies have not worked for you, maybe it's time to question conventional wisdom. Keith did. Here's his story.

Keith knew how the human body worked. He was a chemistry major in college, and he furthered his education to become a chiropractor and certified functional medicine practitioner. By the age of 56, he had spent 25 years in clinical practice. Patients routinely asked him for his recommendations on how to lose weight. Like most doctors, he would share the conventional wisdom to reduce their calorie intake and exercise more, but he knew in the back of his mind that despite their best efforts, his patients had little chance of reaching their weight-loss goal. He knew this from both clinical and personal experience. Despite many attempts to obtain the fit, lean body that he desired, Keith had been overweight since graduating college.

Over the years, he made many wholehearted attempts to lose weight. As an avid exerciser, he rarely missed a week without visits to the gym and often played recreational hockey in an over-35 league. The exercise helped him maintain his lean mass but did not turn the tide on his weight. At one point, he performed an 8-week juice fast that involved consuming nothing but freshly juiced vegetables and fruit three times a day.

> *"He gave it a try, and from that day forward, he found new resolve and tremendous success. IF allowed him to keep the hearty foods that he craved in his diet as long as he cut out sugar, ate more vegetables to give volume to his diet, and declared a time each night to stop eating."*

The juice fast worked, allowing him to shed 43 pounds. But this Midwestern boy who grew up on hearty, meat-based meals could not continue to drink juice and nothing but juice for the rest of his life. As soon as he returned to a nonliquid diet, the pounds returned. And, like many of us, he made countless attempts to follow his own advice, which was to eat fewer calories. A few times a year, he would cut out the hearty meals he loved in exchange for five to six small meals that were, in his view, also small in flavor. Each attempt would allow him to drop a few pounds, but the lack of satisfaction he was experiencing with his food choices would eventually bring the diet to an end. By the age of 56, he had reached his highest weight and was miserable.

Keith's struggle to lose weight didn't only affect him, but it was also hard for his wife and daughter to watch. Because of his weight, Keith snored loudly, so he would often sleep on the couch as not to disturb his wife. His snoring was intense, and as he looks back, it was likely marked by sleep apnea, which is a condition punctuated by periodic stops in breathing. Indeed, his loud snoring was intermixed with periods of unusual quietness that indicated that breathing had momentarily ceased. When his daughter got her first job, she became the first member of the household to get up in the morning. She confessed to her dad that she was fearful of coming down the stairs to find he had died overnight due to his poor health. His wife of 23 years was trying to come to terms with Keith's poor health. It was painful for her to watch him try so hard to lose weight only to be met with yet another failure. One night she professed to him that she had accepted the fact that this man that she loved so dearly might not be with her as long as she had hoped. That statement proved to be the last straw for Keith.

Intermittent fasting was a remote strategy he'd heard of on podcasts, and he had nothing to lose because it was so simple. He gave it a try, and from that day forward, he found new resolve and tremendous success. IF allowed him to keep the hearty foods that he craved in his diet as long as he cut out sugar, ate more vegetables to give volume to his diet, and declared a time each night to stop eating. (By the way, you'll learn this same strategy in Chapter 6.)

Committing to these daily healthy habits provided a glimmer of hope for Keith. For the first time in a long time, he was starting to see that the secret to his *success was to fill his stomach and then take periods to stop eating. Inspired by his new revelation, he started to seek out researchers who were willing to look outside the confines of conventional dietary standards and who were bold enough to ask questions like "If the standard diet recommendations are the best path to health and weight management, why is our society so sick and fat?" With each podcast he'd listen to and research paper he would read, his confidence grew.*

Eating hearty, satisfying meals in a shortened number of hours was easy for him to do; Keith had never been a fan of eating breakfast because he rarely felt hungry in the morning. (Before IF, he would force down a quick breakfast on most mornings because he had bought into the dogma that breakfast is the most important meal of the day.) His new strategy was to skip breakfast and stop eating after dinner. IF was a strategy that fit his lifestyle to a T.

Not only did he see results on the scale, but outward signs of poor health like the swelling in his legs were also going away. On top of that, his snoring had completely vanished, allowing him to gain a reprieve from his exile to the living room couch. For Keith, and many other success stories that you'll be introduced to in this book, intermittent fasting had the stickiness factor needed to turn his health around. The pounds came off, and because he could still eat the hearty meals that he had grown to love, he never went back to his old ways.

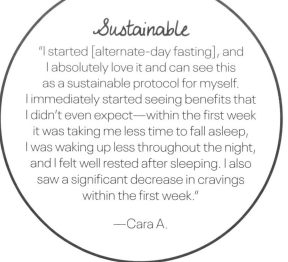

Sustainable

"I started [alternate-day fasting], and I absolutely love it and can see this as a sustainable protocol for myself. I immediately started seeing benefits that I didn't even expect—within the first week it was taking me less time to fall asleep, I was waking up less throughout the night, and I felt well rested after sleeping. I also saw a significant decrease in cravings within the first week."

—Cara A.

By the time 8 months had passed, his weight had dropped by 80 pounds (36kg). He has maintained that weight loss to this day. I know this because Keith, whose full name is Keith Gillaspy, has been my wonderful husband since 1993. After watching his miraculous health turnaround and learning the science of how fasting improves health, I now also practice intermittent fasting most days of the week.

As we move through the book, you'll learn why fasting works for weight loss and be introduced to the science behind how it improves health conditions like diabetes and cardiovascular disease. These benefits are not exclusive to fasting. Many healthy diets boast of improvements in health, and the mere act of losing weight lowers your risk of many diseases. None of this matters, though, if you can't stick with the plan you're on.

WHY WE QUIT DIETS

Behavioral researchers have often pondered the question of why we don't do what we know is good for us. We all know the drill. We should not smoke, we should keep our weight in check, and we should get regular physical activity. We know that fruits and vegetables have vitamins and minerals that support our bodies and that it's important to get adequate sleep at night. These are not earth-shattering health revelations. Most of us have been aware of these health concepts since grade school. So why do so few of us actually do them?

At a symposium held in 2007, a panel of doctors dug deep into what makes us tick with the goal of determining how to improve compliance with routine healthy habits so we could have a healthier society. They found that our collective lack of compliance was not due to a single, glaring issue, but rather a multitude of factors that shape our thoughts about health and ultimately our actions. These influential factors ranged from long-standing social norms to short tidbits of information that flash before our eyes on computer screens or catch our ears as we listen to the radio or talk with friends. All day every day, we are bombarded with diet and lifestyle suggestions that seem to come from every angle. Aunt June swears that her nightly glass of red wine is the secret to her longevity and is constantly badgering you to imbibe with her. Bob from work is a supplement guru who always shares what he's learned and why you need to be taking this, that, and the other thing. The TV commercial tells you that milk does your body good, but the blog you just read says that dairy is bad for you. In essence, what the panel found was that we are suffering from information overload.[1] With so much confusing and conflicting information out there, many of us throw our hands up in frustration and tell the waiter to bring the large pizza with extra cheese as we vow to worry about our health tomorrow.

The symposium doctors uncovered many obstacles we face as we try to live healthy lives, but they also outlined some solutions:

1. **People will change a habit if the change is something they can carry out without complicating their lives.** Complex plans that take over our lives are too much for most of us to comply with, and before long, we end up going back to our old, comfortable routine.

2. **The healthy habits we adopt will stick if they are enjoyed and not dreaded.** The simple truth is that we don't keep doing the things that make us miserable.

3. **We stick with healthy lifestyle choices when we see continual evidence that our plan is working.** Positive results are a great motivator.

Dr. Beckyism

The simple solutions are the best solutions because they are the ones that you'll do.

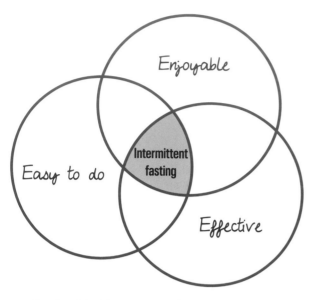

People stick with intermittent fasting because it fulfills the three E's.

Intermittent fasting is best thought of as the cycling of your daily eating pattern between periods of eating (commonly referred to as your *eating window*) and periods of fasting (referred to as your *fasting window*). In scientific literature, this daily eating pattern is often called time-restricted eating and follows this basic formula:

Time-restricted eating

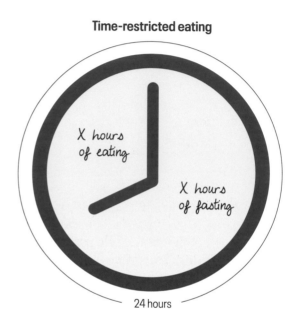

In other words, for you to stick with healthy habits that will lead to better health and weight loss, you need to create a plan that is easy to do, enjoyable, and effective. I call these my three E's, and intermittent fasting fulfills them all.

It's Easy to Do

Fasting is nothing new. People have been practicing it for millennia for religious reasons or as a way of cleansing the body of impurities. Yet, in our modern world of confusing diets and conflicting information, it is truly revolutionary in its simplicity.

As we move through the book, I will introduce you to different intermittent fasting strategies so you can find one that fits your lifestyle. I'll discuss fasting variations like every-other-day fasts and extended fasts.

Have you ever been on a diet and felt like you had to vigilantly remember to eat at precise times or to meticulously record your combination of nutrients? I'm not saying that fine-tuning your diet is a worthless pursuit. In fact, I'll go over good nutritional choices in later chapters. I am simply saying that with fasting, you can breathe a sigh of relief. There are no complicated hoops to jump through. To perform a fast, you note the time of day, stop eating, and then start again when your fast is complete.

You'll also love the flexibility that you have with intermittent fasting. You don't even have to do the same fasting routine every day to reap the benefits. Do you have a breakfast meeting on Wednesday? That's fine; go ahead and have breakfast, lunch, and dinner that day. Do you have a busy morning on Thursday? Save time by skipping breakfast and just eat lunch and dinner. Before long, you will find your groove and do what feels right for your body.

By this point, you're likely suspecting that there may also be a simplistic explanation for why intermittent fasting and weight loss are linked. Plainly stated, when you don't take in calories, you don't gain weight.

Indeed, many of the intermittent fasting studies performed on humans show that reducing the number of hours during which we eat naturally lends itself to a lower caloric intake for the entire day. It is logical to conclude that this observation is part of the reason why periods of fasting are useful for weight loss. Earlier in the book, I mentioned a study on breakfast skippers who, although they ate more calories at lunchtime, never made up for those calories in the remaining hours of the day (see page 18). By day's end, they had a net reduction in their daily calorie intake. Many intermittent fasting strategies also naturally reduce late-night snacking and alcohol consumption. These factors could contribute to the natural caloric restriction and weight loss associated with fasting.[2] This unconscious reduction in calories has led some researchers to speculate that a reason for intermittent fasting's growing popularity is because people find it easier to follow than traditional calorie-restricted diets.[3]

There's no doubt that *not* eating is a pretty easy concept for most of us to absorb, but eating is fun. How could fasting possibly fulfill the enjoyable component of the three E's?

It's Enjoyable

The thing to keep in mind is that intermittent fasting is a way of changing your eating pattern rather than a diet that dictates food choices. That doesn't mean you can eat cheeseburgers, candy bars, and milkshakes throughout a shortened eating window and expect better health and weight loss. It does mean, however, that intermittent fasting enhances the benefits of all types of healthy diets, from a well-formulated vegan diet to a well-formulated keto diet. Are you not a meat eater? You don't have to compromise this ideal to benefit from intermittent fasting. Are you more like my husband, a Midwestern guy who wouldn't want to live without his hearty, meal-based meals? You, too, can gain benefits from IF without fundamentally changing your diet preference.

Simplified meal planning

"I find this method of eating is becoming increasingly easy. I began with fasting 12:12 and have now lengthened to 16:8 at least twice a week. As time has progressed, I find the fasting is getting much easier and it really simplifies meal planning! I have about 8lbs to go before I reach my goal, but I believe I will set a lower goal."

— Colleen H.

Ultimately there is nothing more enjoyable in life than having good health. One of the best aspects of intermittent fasting is that it comes with so many great perks above and beyond weight loss. Many people experience mental clarity and better focus when they fast and report that they feel great during the fast. Who knew?! Not to mention, it's just pure fun to step on the scale and see that your weight has gone down.

All of these perks come with the satisfaction of being able to eat with your family and friends, even if they aren't on your diet. Intermittent fasting gives you a break from having to cook two dinners: one for the family and one that meets your diet requirements. You can partake at company functions without standing out. ("Oh boy, it looks like Shirley's on another diet.") Yes, I know that we should not worry about what other people say about us, but we've all been in those situations where we felt that all eyes were upon us. With intermittent fasting, there is a measure of anonymity, and whether it's right or wrong, there's peace in that understanding for many of us.

I'd be remiss if I did not mention a final endearing aspect of intermittent fasting, which is that it is a true time- and money-saver. It takes no time and no money to prepare no food.

Dr. Beckyism

Others might question why you have changed your eating habits, but there is no need to defend something that works. Results speak louder and clearer than your words ever can.

It's Effective

Intermittent fasting gives you the flexibility and freedom to eat your preferred type of diet, all while saving time and money; those are some pretty impressive attributes. However, they mean little if they do not produce the health and weight-loss benefits you desire. You think "If I'm going to put the effort in, then show me the results!" To understand how fasting produces these benefits, let's look at how your body processes the food you eat and what happens when you don't eat.

We tend to overlook the fact that we all fast on a daily basis. We just call it sleep. During the day, we periodically take in food, providing the raw materials that our bodies convert to energy. Some of that energy gets used right away, and some gets tucked away in storage for later use. When you sleep, your body pulls from that stored energy to perform important functions such as keeping your heart beating and your lungs breathing. It is a pretty slick operation, and your body is perfectly equipped to handle the hours when no food is coming in.

In a way, intermittent fasting is like a form of biohacking, or intentionally manipulating your lifestyle (your eating schedule) to affect your biology and achieve a desired state. It puts *you* in control!

- By cycling periods of eating with periods of fasting, you put your body into periods of enhanced fat burning.

- Fasting keeps your blood sugar level low, which is an anti-inflammatory state that is good for your health and specific blood sugar–related problems like insulin resistance and diabetes.

- Fasting gives your body welcome time off from the exhausting process of digesting food, which frees up resources for other operations like *autophagy*. Autophagy is a housekeeping process that your body performs to remove or recycle unneeded or damaged cellular components.

- Not eating close to bedtime allows time for your core body temperature to drop, which helps you sleep more soundly.

Intermittent fasting is easy to do, enjoyable, and effective. With its many benefits, IF seems like a health hack that everyone should be doing. The next chapter further elaborates on the many health benefits of fasting, as well as the basic science of how your body converts food to energy.

WHO SHOULD—AND SHOULD NOT—FAST?

Health is a very individualized thing, so before we dive into the "how-to" of fasting, we need to stop and ask the question "Is fasting right for you?"

Are you taking a medication?

As a rule, anytime you are thinking about changing your diet or eating pattern, you should let your doctor know about your intentions. This rule of thumb is particularly important for people taking medications, especially if the medications are to be taken with food or for conditions that can be influenced by your diet, including, but not limited to, diabetes and cardiovascular-related issues.[4]

Do you have a history of an eating disorder or being underweight?

Past health history and body composition are also factors to consider when deciding if fasting is right for you. For instance, fasting would be ill-advised for those with a history of an eating disorder or those who are currently underweight or in a frail or weakened state. For these subsets of individuals, proper nutrition is important, so the restriction of food or calories is not recommended.

Are you pregnant or breastfeeding?

Women who are pregnant or breastfeeding should not fast. Nutrition is vital for a developing fetus so it can grow and thrive within the womb. A breastfed baby obtains all of their nutrients from Mom, so nutritional care should continue after giving birth. I am not suggesting that fasting will cause a pregnant or breastfeeding mother to suffer from malnutrition, but this is not a time of life to experiment with your eating routine. Pregnancy and breastfeeding are two unique periods in a woman's life, and although fasting is not recommended for those times, it doesn't preclude her from using fasting at other times in her life. If a woman is looking to become pregnant, it is wise to consult with her doctor before embarking on a fasting routine.

Is fasting safe for women?

During a woman's reproductive years, the main safety concern is that calorie intake does not drop to a point where the young woman's menstrual cycle could be disrupted.

To date, much of the research that has been done on the effects of fasting on a young female body has been done on rodents. Animal research is valuable because it provides clues, but obvious limitations exist when trying to translate the results to humans. What has been revealed is that longer-term fasts, such as full-day fasting or other regimens that cause a large calorie deficit, may disrupt the menstrual cycle.[5, 6]

An observational study of teenage girls who fasted during Ramadan found that regular fasting caused changes in girls' menstrual cycles, especially in menstrual blood volume.[7] However, these types of studies rely on self-reporting and inference, leaving many questions unanswered. Because of the complex hormonal changes that come with puberty and the lack of research that exists, fasting would not be advisable for a teenage girl, particularly at the onset of puberty.

Other women of reproductive age will do best to look at short-term fasting routines that do not result in large calorie deficits. Regardless of age, it is important for women to eat well during their eating window to ensure proper nutrition.

Aside from the cautions mentioned earlier, the scientific literature has revealed that fasting, when done wisely, is a safe practice for pre- and post-menopausal women of normal health. A research team dug through the scientific literature looking for studies related to fasting, women's health, and women's disorders. They found that fasting had numerous benefits for women, including improvements in reproductive as well as mental health, which was revealed as a decrease in anxiety and depression and improvements in mood.

The review also found that fasting was effective in reducing belly fat. Managing belly fat is important to women of all ages, but particularly important for post-menopausal women. Increased belly fat contributes to a condition called *metabolic syndrome,* which is a collection of health issues that increases a post-menopausal woman's risk of cardiovascular disease and diabetes. Fasting was found to combat metabolic syndrome, which would have an overall heart-protective effect for women as they age.

The benefits did not stop there. The research team also found evidence that fasting may aid in the treatment of certain cancers, improve bone health, and reduce inflammation in the body, which is an underlying condition in many chronic diseases. The research team concluded that although there is a need for large, well-designed studies on women and fasting, "fasting can be prescribed as a safe medical intervention as well as a lifestyle regimen which can improve women's health in many folds."[8]

Is fasting safe for children?

Women and men of normal health have the green light to fast, but what about kids? This question does not have a clear answer. What we do know is that a child's body uses calories for growth, so it is possible that a child benefits from eating three meals stretched throughout the day. Studies that are available on children reveal that preschool children who regularly eat breakfast weigh less than those who skip breakfast, and school-aged children do better in school when they eat in the morning.[9, 10] However, studies like these rely on things like surveys and observations to draw their conclusions. It is not realistic to perform controlled studies on children that would require them to fast so that we can determine if fasting is harmful. Without that more conclusive look, we can't be certain that the positive results we see in young breakfast eaters are due to the breakfast itself or other factors that they might have in common.

MORE IS NOT NECESSARILY BETTER

I want to leave you with one last thought before we move on: fasting is great, but more is not necessarily better. It is true that even a lean person carries around a lot of spare energy. Glycogen (stored sugar) accounts for a small amount of this energy reserve (about 2,000 calories' worth), but with every pound of fat estimated to contain around 3,500 calories of energy, even a lean person may have tens of thousands of calories to burn.

If you are overweight, you might be wondering that if fasting for half of the day is good, wouldn't half of the month be better? Certainly, people have gone long periods without food, but good health is a balance. If you have a thought brewing in your head that you are just going to stop eating until you reach your goal, I urge you to reconsider. There is no point in losing weight if you are also losing your health.

You want to make sure that you are providing your body with the nutrients it needs to perform at its best. This book is about fasting, but it is also a diet guide. I encourage you to use the information in Part 2 to optimize your food intake as you intersperse periods of fasting.

3

THE SCIENCE OF FASTING

What lies ahead

- **Excess insulin causes your body to store fat.** Fasting keeps insulin levels low, allowing your body to shift to a fat-burning state so you can lose weight.

- **Fasting has a multiplicity of health benefits beyond losing weight.** It can improve brain function, reduce cardiovascular stress, promote autophagy, lower blood sugar, decrease inflammation, improve gut health, and make your metabolism more adaptable.

- **There is a tipping point during fasting when you will start to lose muscle.** However, the body typically will not burn lean tissue until a fast exceeds about 24 hours.

Social media is filled with anecdotal claims of better health and weight loss through intermittent fasting, but can these claims be backed up by the scientific literature? In this chapter, you'll discover what happens inside of your body when you fast and how fasting enhances the metabolic processes that allow you to take control of your health and weight.

FOOD IS ENERGY

The energy contained in food is what we refer to as *calories*. Your heart, lungs, and other organs don't run on food energy (calories); they run on body energy (or technically stated, a compound called *ATP—adenosine triphosphate*). In other words, the food you eat must get digested and turned into simple molecules that your cells can take in and convert to ATP. Three main food nutrients contain calories; they are carbohydrates, proteins, and fats. Collectively, we call them *macronutrients*. Foods also contain vitamins and minerals, which are referred to as *micronutrients*. Micronutrients support your metabolism and health, but because they don't have calories, they don't directly supply energy like their macronutrient counterparts.

Your digestive tract is the first stop for the macronutrients. Here, the carbs, proteins, and fats are met by enzymes and digestive juices that go to work breaking them into their basic elements: sugar (glucose), amino acids, and fatty acids, respectively.

Most whole foods have a combination of the three macronutrients. For instance, nuts and seeds provide your body with all three macronutrients, while beans and other legumes contain little fat but supply your system with a mix of carbs and protein. Meat, fish, and eggs contain protein and fat but minuscule amounts of carbs. I appreciate the fact that learning which foods contain which nutrients can make your head spin; the meal plans provided in the second part of this book have been broken down into their nutrient profiles, so you don't have to worry about memorizing these facts. However, having an overview of how your body handles different nutrients will help you better understand how fasting benefits you.

Fast fact: a quick macronutrient trick

A quick trick for telling if a food contains carbohydrates is to think about its source. Did it come from an animal or a plant? The source of a food matters because plants are the living organisms that make carbohydrates. Photosynthesis is a process by which plants use sunlight, carbon dioxide, and water to make glucose (a carbohydrate). Therefore, all plant foods contain carbs. Most animal-based foods contain only trace amounts of carbs, with the exception being some dairy, which contains a type of sugar called lactose.

Carbs, Glucose, and Insulin

The word *carbohydrate* can be used to describe a multitude of foods. Some of them have health benefits (vegetables, fruits, whole grains, and beans), while the consumption of other carbs (sugar-sweetened drinks, white bread, pasta, and the three C's—cookies, cakes, and candies) have been linked with health consequences. Once a carb breaks down into a simple glucose molecule, it can easily pass into your bloodstream. Your bloodstream is under tight controls, and doesn't like to have too much glucose floating through it at any given time. To move excess glucose out of your blood, your pancreas pumps out a hormone called insulin. When everything is working as it should, insulin opens the doors to your cells, which gladly accept it and use it to make ATP. If there is no immediate need for energy, the glucose molecules can be linked together and stored as glycogen in your muscles or liver. When these storage sites get filled, your liver can convert glucose into fat that can be stored in your adipose (fat) tissue.

Protein and Amino Acids

Your body likes to turn the carbs you eat into energy, but protein is used differently. Instead of being used as a primary energy source, protein goes through an interesting recycling process within your body. When protein molecules meet the digestive juices, they get broken down into amino acids and head to your bloodstream, following a similar path to that of glucose. However, unlike glucose, whose primary job is to become energy, amino acids are used to make new body proteins. Amino acids would be expensive fuel because they have so many other important uses. When your cells take in amino acids, they use them to assemble new proteins that are needed by the cells. Does your thyroid need more thyroid hormone? Your thyroid cells take up amino acids and use them to make thyroid hormones. Do you need to replenish liver enzymes? That requires amino acids. Have you been working out at the gym? Amino acids are the building blocks of muscle. This is not to say that protein cannot be used as energy, and indeed this can happen with severe caloric restriction and long fasts (more on this on pages 47–49), but you can see that burning amino acids as a main fuel source would be a waste of a valuable commodity.

How do carbs (glucose) become body fat?

You eat some **carbs** →

1. If your body needs energy right now to complete a function, your cells will first use the glucose to create ATP (usable body energy). If energy is not needed, or if there is still glucose left over, then...

2. Your body links the available glucose together and stores it as glycogen in your muscles and liver. If your glycogen stores are full and you still have glucose remaining, then...

3. Your body turns the remaining glucose into fat and stores it in your adipose tissue until it's needed.

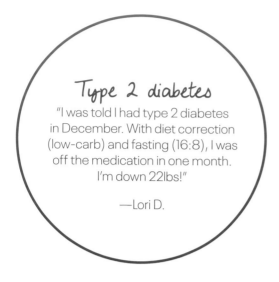

Fats and Fatty Acids

Dietary fats are found in whole foods like meat, dairy, fish, eggs, nuts, and seeds. They are also found in processed meats and snack foods, as well as pure fat sources like oil and butter. Dietary fats enter your digestive tract as relatively large fat globs. Those large globs get broken down into smaller fat globules by a substance called bile. When the globules are small enough, they get acted upon by enzymes that continue to help with their breakdown. The fat you eat requires a few extra steps before entering your bloodstream because, unlike carbs and proteins, fats don't like water. Because your bloodstream is a watery environment, fatty acids must put on a special coat before passing into the lining of your digestive tract and making their way into your blood as a watertight molecule known as a *chylomicron*. As the chylomicron circulates, it can drop off its fatty cargo in places like muscles and adipose tissues where it can be used as immediate energy or stored for later use.

The "Cost" of Energy

To further your understanding of how your body uses the three macros for energy, let's use an analogy. Think of your body as a bank. When you deposit money into a bank, the bank converts the paper money into an electronic record so it can be stored on their computer. To perform that task, the bank charges you a fee, which decreases the amount of your balance. When you want to buy something, you withdraw money from your balance.

A similar sequence of events happens inside of your body as you cycle between eating and fasting. When you deposit food calories into your body, it converts them into stored energy (i.e., glycogen or fat). However, not all of the energy gets stored—some is burned immediately and disappears, much like the fee amount that your bank took. When you want to do something active or when you're fasting, your body dips into the balance of energy stored in glycogen and fat.

Another thing to consider with the banking analogy is that unlike when you visit the bank, where you can do multiple transactions per visit, your body prefers a one-transaction-per-visit policy. You are either depositing energy or withdrawing it. When you eat, energy gets stored. When you don't eat (i.e., fast), energy is released.

The conductor of this storage-and-release symphony is insulin, which you can think of as your fat-storing hormone. When insulin is elevated in your blood, your body is in fat-storing mode. When it is low, your body is in fat-burning mode. Insulin levels rise when you eat. When you fast, insulin levels drop.

WEIGHT GAIN/LOSS AND INSULIN

To appreciate how fasting helps you lose weight, it's helpful to understand how weight gain happens. Insulin plays a key role in the sculpting of body fat. When insulin is high, you store fat, and when it's low, you release fat. This knowledge might give you the impression that insulin is a bad character you'd be better off without. In reality, you couldn't live without insulin and its fat-storing ability. Although it is sometimes hard to imagine, body fat is important! Without a way to store energy for later use, you could not survive. However, adipose tissue is a seemingly endless storage closet. If it grows too big, it becomes uncomfortable, impedes activity, creates inflammation, and promotes disease.

Insulin is the hormone that helps fill our fat cells, but we can't blame insulin for the weight epidemic that has hit our society and led to obesity rates exceeding 35 percent of the U.S. population.[1] Insulin is merely doing its job. It would be like blaming the mail carrier for an overstuffed mailbox. Insulin, like the mail carrier, is just delivering the goods. If we want to prevent the overstuffing of our fat cells, we need to eat in a way that gives insulin less to do. That's not easy to do in our modern world of abundance.

Unlike our ancestors, we have 24/7 access to food, so insulin is continually called into work. Many of the foods available to us have been altered from their natural state to increase their shelf life and crave factor. Our bodies digest and absorb these refined foods quickly, which requires insulin to spike as it deals with the rapid influx of nutrients.

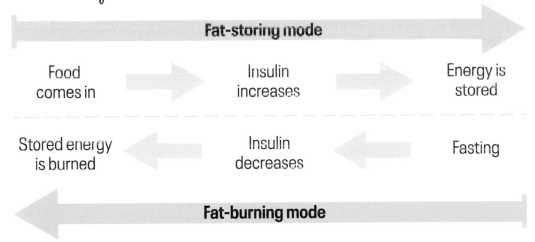

The role of insulin

Fat-storing mode

Food comes in → Insulin increases → Energy is stored

Stored energy is burned ← Insulin decreases ← Fasting

Fat-burning mode

Fasting gives your body a break from producing insulin to regulate blood sugar. This tells your body that it should tap into fat stores or glycogen for fuel.

These processed and refined foods are calorie-dense, which helps explain why the average person's daily calorie consumption has increased by 24 percent since 1960s.[2] In other words, we've gained weight because of abundance and excess. To lose weight, some restrictions must occur. What we choose to cut back on is up to us.

Dr. Beckyism

When you eat sugar, you get a spike in your blood sugar, which spikes the fat-storing hormone insulin. Long story short, sugar is a great food for making you fat.

There are three different ways to approach losing weight: (1) limiting certain foods (fats, carbs, or refined foods), (2) limiting how much you eat (calories), or (3) limiting the number of hours during which you consume food (intermittent fasting). Traditional weight-loss methods have focused on the first two options, and there is certainly evidence that cutting back on calories or reducing your intake of refined and processed foods works for weight loss, regardless of whether you follow a low-fat or low-carb lifestyle.[3, 4]

The third option, fasting, is an ancient tradition that has long been thought to have physical and spiritual healing properties, but its use as a weight-loss tool is fairly recent. The time you spend fasting frees insulin of its workload, putting your body in a state that favors fat burning. Fasting also naturally reduces calories by eliminating high-caloric habits like eating refined snacks at bedtime and consuming alcohol in the evening. So fasting provides two weight-loss advantages right off the bat—lower insulin and reduced calories. Because you are restricting time rather than food, you can pair it with a healthy diet to give your body fat a one-two punch. Let's look more into the weight loss and health advantages by learning what happens inside your body when you fast.

THE BIOLOGICAL BENEFITS OF INTERMITTENT FASTING

Your body views periods of fasting as good stress. When you lift weights at the gym, you put stress on your muscles. Your muscles respond to this good stress by getting stronger. Your body undergoes a similar stress-strengthening reaction when you fast. This positive stress reaction is referred to as *hormesis* (i.e., what doesn't kill you makes you stronger). Hormesis triggers a host of adaptive responses that protect your cells, repair damage, and strengthen metabolic pathways and processes.

Never hungry!

"IF has absolutely helped me. I lost 80lbs/6 dress sizes and have kept it off for several years. I eat all of my calories every day (following no diet or eating diet foods). I'm never hungry. It has helped me to stop the after-dinner snacking, and in general I've learned how to have a healthier relationship with food. Also, I love eating bigger meals and not going over my maintenance calories. I don't ever see myself going back to eating snacks and small meals all day."

—Alisha

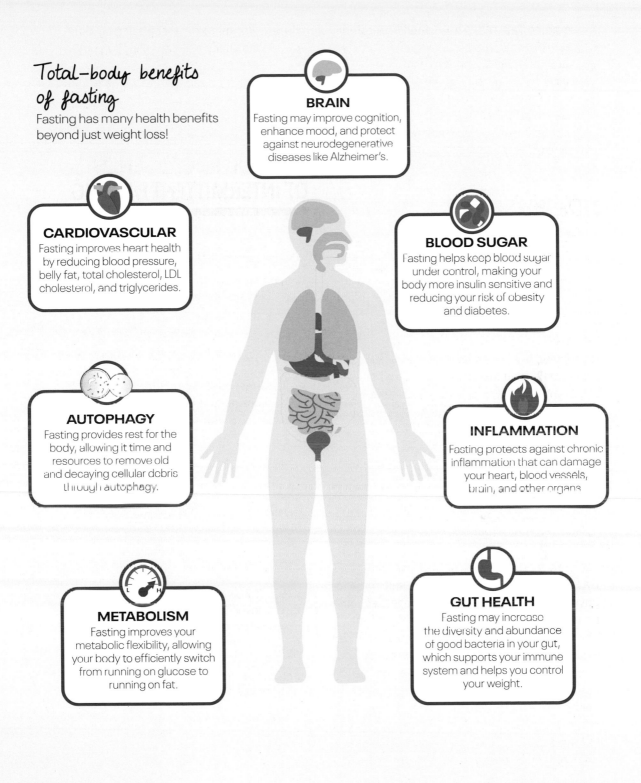

Total-body benefits of fasting

Fasting has many health benefits beyond just weight loss!

BRAIN
Fasting may improve cognition, enhance mood, and protect against neurodegenerative diseases like Alzheimer's.

CARDIOVASCULAR
Fasting improves heart health by reducing blood pressure, belly fat, total cholesterol, LDL cholesterol, and triglycerides.

BLOOD SUGAR
Fasting helps keep blood sugar under control, making your body more insulin sensitive and reducing your risk of obesity and diabetes.

AUTOPHAGY
Fasting provides rest for the body, allowing it time and resources to remove old and decaying cellular debris through autophagy.

INFLAMMATION
Fasting protects against chronic inflammation that can damage your heart, blood vessels, brain, and other organs.

METABOLISM
Fasting improves your metabolic flexibility, allowing your body to efficiently switch from running on glucose to running on fat.

GUT HEALTH
Fasting may increase the diversity and abundance of good bacteria in your gut, which supports your immune system and helps you control your weight.

Not only are you making your body more resilient through fasting, but you are also giving it a break. During fasting, your body gets time off from the energy-demanding process of digesting food. This rest period provides your body the time it needs to tend to general housekeeping tasks and restock substances necessary for maintenance and repair. Think of fasting as a restaurant after hours. When the restaurant is full of customers, the workers are busy serving food and there's no time to clean up or restock the shelves. When the restaurant closes and the customers have all gone, the staff has time to complete their chores. Let's look at just how much the body can accomplish when it is not preoccupied with food.

Improved Blood Sugar Control to Lower Diabetes Risk

Blood sugar and *insulin* are words that we associate with diabetes. What if you don't have that condition? Should you care that fasting controls blood sugar and insulin levels? Yes! I already mentioned that chronically high insulin levels keep your body locked in fat-storing mode. But for insulin to climb, there needs to be a trigger. The biggest trigger is the presence of sugar in the blood. Think of insulin as a fire hose and sugar as a fire in your bloodstream. If there is a big fire, a lot of water is needed to put out the flames. Likewise, when there is a lot of sugar in your blood, a lot of insulin is needed to return your blood sugar level to normal.

The standard American diet (appropriately nicknamed SAD) is a diet high in blood sugar–spiking refined carbohydrates (think pizza, pasta, bread, and cookies). As we learned in Chapter 1, many of us are all-day grazers, consuming these unhealthy foods with few breaks from sun up to sundown. The continual blood sugar and insulin spikes that result encourage weight gain, which contributes to the onset of blood sugar disorders like prediabetes and diabetes.[5, 6] The spikes are followed by blood sugar crashes that drive hunger and cravings.

IF is a way of disrupting the progression of blood sugar disorders and controlling hunger. With no food coming in, there is no rise in blood sugar or insulin. This downtime is beneficial in different ways:

- A study involving eight prediabetic men showed that following an early time-restricted eating schedule improved the body's response to insulin. The men consumed all of their calories for the day within a 6-hour eating window, with their final meal ending before 3pm. At the end of the study, the men saw improvements in insulin sensitivity as well as the function of their pancreas, which is the organ that produces insulin.[7]

- A clinical study found that eating within a 10-hour window may help stave off diabetes by reducing metabolic syndrome, which is a cluster of conditions, including chronically high blood sugar, high blood pressure, high triglycerides, increased belly fat, and low HDL cholesterol.[8]

- It has been postulated that the rest the body receives from routine fasting may reset cellular sensitivity, making it easier for your cells to respond to insulin and glucose and lowering your risk of developing diabetes.[9]

Fast fact: fighting cancer

Cancer is a complex topic. There are multiple forms of cancer, each with unanswered questions about its cause and progression. Therefore, science is far from stating that fasting cures cancer. However, this is an area of exciting research. Lab studies performed on mice and cells show that cycles of fasting may delay the progression of certain tumors and increase the effectiveness of cancer treatments like chemotherapy and radiation.[10, 11, 12] Although human studies are few and far between, some interesting research involving women with breast cancer has emerged. In a study led by researcher Catherine Marinac, it was discovered that fasting 13 or more hours per night lowered a woman's risk of breast cancer recurrence by as much as 36 percent.[13]

- The improved insulin sensitivity and blood sugar regulation that is achieved through fasting prevents the dips in blood sugar that drive cravings, making it easier to stretch out the time between meals.

Reduced Inflammation to Boost Overall Health

Chronically high blood sugar creates an inflammatory state in your body. Inflammation is something you want to happen when you have a cut on your skin or you're fighting off an infection. When these things happen, the inflammatory process helps clear out damage and heal the tissue.

When the job of healing is complete, the inflammation goes away. However, some lifestyle factors, such as smoking, obesity, and chronic stress, hold your body in a constant state of inflammation. This prolonged state can cause damage to your heart, blood vessels, brain, and other organs.

IF encourages positive cellular responses and activates pathways that enhance internal defenses against inflammation.[10] The side benefit of not eating late into the evening may contribute to the inflammation-lowering effect that is seen with fasting. In a study on women from the 2009–2010 National Health and Nutrition Examination Survey (NHANES), researchers found that each 10 percent increase in the proportion of calories eaten after 5pm resulted in a 3 percent increase in inflammation. The finding suggests that reducing food intake at night and fasting for longer nightly intervals may lower inflammation in the body.[14]

Boosted Metabolism and Metabolic Flexibility

When you fast, your body is provided with the time and rest it needs to create chemical and hormonal advantages that boost metabolism. Your metabolism is the sum total of all the chemical processes going on inside your body. Certain regulators of metabolism, such as norepinephrine and growth hormone (GH), are increased through fasting.[15, 16] Norepinephrine levels naturally drop when you go to bed. As the sun comes up, so does your level of norepinephrine, making it a part of the cocktail of chemicals that wakes you up and prepares your body and brain for activity. Growth hormone, as its name suggests, is a hormone that helps you grow. GH is obviously important in youth, but it's also still useful in adulthood by helping to regulate metabolism and muscle mass.[17] As you move through your adult years, levels of GH naturally decrease, which can lead to the onset of frailty as you age. Therefore, the more secretion of GH that you can encourage, the better. One way to do this is through fasting. The secretion of GH is suppressed when you are in a fed state, and it is enhanced when you are in a fasted state, which is why fasting has been shown to boost levels of GH in adults.[16]

Not only does fasting help your body keep metabolically important hormones high, it also makes you more metabolically flexible. In a nutshell, *metabolic flexibility* means your body can adapt to the fuel source that is most readily available. Earlier in the chapter, I mentioned that your body gets calories from macronutrients (carbs, fats, and protein). Your body breaks down those nutrients into their basic forms (glucose, fatty acids, and amino acids) so they can be burned for immediate energy or stored to meet future energy needs. Your body's favorite energy-storage sites are glycogen (stored glucose) and adipose tissue (stored fatty acids). When you eat all day long without intentional calorie restriction, the nutrients that you take in meet the energy needs of your body. With its energy demand satisfied, there is no reason for your body to go to the trouble of pulling fuel out of storage. So constant feeding makes you rather metabolically inflexible. Your body happily runs on the glucose coming in from your diet. If it needs a bit more energy, it taps into the easy-to-access glycogen stored in your liver (a source much easier to access than fat).

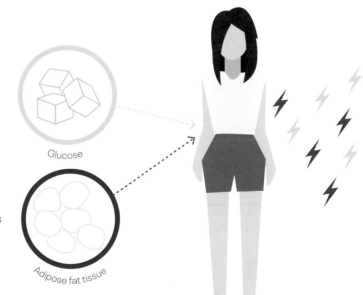

Metabolic flexibility

This is when your body has the effortless ability to switch between using glucose and fat as fuel. Fasting increases your metabolic flexibility, allowing your body to use the fuel source that is most readily available.

Glucose

Adipose fat tissue

Fast fact: fasting and your brain

Could fasting help you think more clearly, improve your mood, or protect you from neurodegenerative disorders like Alzheimer's disease? As of this date, most of the research in these areas has been done on rodents, but the research is encouraging:

- Studies have shown that alternate-day fasting results in improved motor coordination and cognitive skills and enhanced learning and memory.[19, 20]

- A review of the scientific literature revealed that fasting is often associated with improved mood. A range of possible mood-enhancing triggers has been identified, from the release of feel-good chemicals in the body and brain, to improved sleep quality, to the production of the brain-fueling ketones that come with fasting.[21]

- According to a study published in the *New England Journal of Medicine,* alternate-day fasting can delay the onset of neurodegenerative diseases in animals. Whether this benefit transfers to humans is yet to be tested.[10]

- Although not focused entirely on fasting, there is evidence that Alzheimer's disease is linked to impairment in glucose metabolism similar to that observed in type 2 diabetics. This link between dementia and diabetes has led some scientists to refer to Alzheimer's as type 3 diabetes.[22] Because fasting is effective in the fight against diabetes, it is logical to think that fasting could delay or prevent the onset of Alzheimer's.

One the other hand, when you fast, you make your body work harder to meet its energy needs. This is a good thing because your body becomes efficient at switching from one fuel source (glucose) to another (fat). In other words, fasting makes you metabolically flexible.

The good news doesn't stop there. Fasting also encourages the production of a third fuel source called ketones. When you fast, no nutrients are coming into your system, so your liver breaks down the glycogen it has tucked away, which provides your body with the glucose it needs to keep running. However, glycogen stores run out rather quickly, so after about 12 to 24 hours (depending on your activity level and energy usage), your body starts to run on fat.[11] Fat is stored in adipose tissue as a molecule called a *triglyceride.* A triglyceride contains three

fatty acids held together by a backbone called *glycerol*. When triglycerides break down, they provide two sources of energy: (1) the newly freed fatty acids and (2) glucose made from the glycerol backbone.

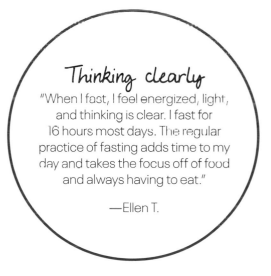

Thinking clearly

"When I fast, I feel energized, light, and thinking is clear. I fast for 16 hours most days. The regular practice of fasting adds time to my day and takes the focus off of food and always having to eat."

—Ellen T.

Brain food!

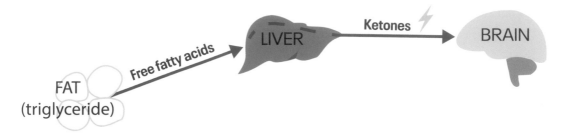

When your body's supply of glycogen (stored glucose) runs low during your fast, your body releases free fatty acids (FFAs) from fat cells. FFAs can be used as direct fuel by many tissues, but not by your brain. To fuel the brain, your liver converts some FFAs to ketones.

Glucose is a universal fuel that can be used by all of your cells. Free fatty acids also act as fuel, but some organs, such as your brain, cannot use them directly. Your brain cells will continue to use glucose for energy, but with glycogen stores depleted and only a small amount of glucose coming from the breakdown of fat, it would seem that you are at the end of the road for fueling the brain. If this were the end of the story, then anyone who fasts would be crippled by brain fog. That is far from the truth, with many people reporting improved mental clarity and mood with fasting (see the *Fast fact* on page 43).

The trick that your body is holding up its sleeve is ketones. Although some fatty acids released from the triglycerides are used directly for fuel, they are in general a poor fuel source for your brain. Instead, the liver processes them to become *ketones,* or ketone bodies.[18] As it turns out, your brain thrives on ketones, which act as a new fuel for your body and brain cells.[11]

You can see that routine fasting puts positive stress on your body that requires it to create new pathways of energy production. You become metabolically flexible as your body switches from its reliance on glucose in a fed state to burning glucose, fatty acids, ketones, and some amino acids (more on this later in the chapter) in a fasted state. This ability to quickly switch from one fuel source to another could account for reports of improved mental clarity and energy in those who fast regularly.

Improved Heart Health, Blood Pressure, and Cholesterol

Most lives do not go untouched by heart disease. Whether we have to deal with it personally or it affects a loved one, most will come face to face with the reality that heart disease is a leading cause of death and can rob people of their quality of their life.[23]

The cardiovascular system is a transport system for your body. Your blood vessels act as the highways, and your heart is the main hub that keeps the system moving. If the highways get clogged, the system breaks down, increasing your risk of heart attack, angina (chest pain), or stroke. What clogs the highways? Plaque. We blame cholesterol for plaque buildup, and plaque indeed contains cholesterol. But putting all the blame on cholesterol for the narrowing of arteries is like blaming a Band-Aid for the cut on your arm. If the cut weren't there in the first place, the Band-Aid would have no reason to be there. Likewise, cholesterol has to have a reason to stick to the vessel wall. One of the primary reasons is chronic inflammation that causes injury to the vessel lining. Think of the redness and swelling that surrounds a cut on your finger and then think of that happening inside of a delicate blood vessel, and you'll appreciate how inflammation increases your risk of cardiovascular disease.

Better blood markers

"After a decade of being significantly overweight with heightened blood sugar, high blood pressure, and high triglyceride levels (nonalcoholic fatty liver disease), I decided to reduce my carb and sugar intake. I was quickly able to reduce my weight [by 20lbs]. I now do IF by eating two meals a day within an 8-hour window. I have maintained my blood sugar, blood pressure, triglyceride levels, and weight at healthier levels for 6 months (and counting)."

—Greg P.

Fortunately, as we learned earlier, IF is effective at lowering inflammation. The reduction of inflammation that comes with fasting is likely part of the reason why intermittent fasting is effective at treating cardiovascular disease. But many other cardiovascular benefits have been linked to fasting:

- **Improved cholesterol profile:** There are good and bad sides to cholesterol. It is a critical component of many hormones and helps form the border around every cell in your body, but too much of the wrong cholesterol has health consequences. So the goal is not to get your total cholesterol down to zero, but rather to have a collection of heart-healthy blood markers, including low total cholesterol, LDL cholesterol, and triglycerides, as well as a high level of HDL cholesterol. IF has been shown to improve these markers.[8, 10, 24, 25]

- **Reduced blood pressure:** Having high blood pressure puts a lot of strain on the blood vessels and heart. The benefits of intermittent fasting for reducing blood pressure are not always reflected in the research. This fact may be because many studies are short term, lasting only a few weeks or months. However, some studies support the premise that IF can reduce blood pressure.[7, 8, 10, 26]

- **Stronger blood vessels:** As we age, our blood vessels are more susceptible to damage. Ketones that are produced during a fast have been found to delay vascular aging of the delicate inner lining of the vessels.[27] Also, fasting may add a layer of protection for the vessel linings through the reduction of oxidative stress.[28]

Oxidative stress is a condition that occurs when the body creates too many cell-damaging molecules called *free radicals*. Free radicals are particularly damaging to the vessel linings.

- **Reduced belly fat:** Having a large waist circumference is one of the components of metabolic syndrome, which is a condition that increases your risk of heart disease, stroke, and type 2 diabetes. I've discussed how fasting is effective for weight loss, but it is particularly helpful in reducing dangerous belly fat.[8, 24]

Fast fact: live longer

Can you live longer on less? It has been shown that continual calorie restriction increases the life span of animals.[36, 37] Although the research has only been done on rodents, we see that intermittent fasting has a similar longevity perk. One study showed that mice that ate one meal a day lived 11 to 14 percent longer than mice fed the same number of calories without time restriction.[38]

Increased Cellular Housekeeping (Autophagy)

Autophagy has a science-y name, but is easy to understand when you break the word down. The first part of the word, *auto*, means "self," and the latter half, *phagia*, means "eating." Autophagy literally means "self-eating," and that is exactly what is happening when this process takes place inside your body. During this housekeeping, your cells eat themselves when they die

of natural causes, they sustain damage, or your body needs the cells' components to make something else, such as energy. You can think of autophagy as a self-cleaning system that is in place to clear out the dead cells and debris that would otherwise pile up. This cleanup is important because decaying cells give off harmful substances called *inflammatory cytokines,* which spread the damage to more cells, much like a rotten apple causes the whole bushel of apples to go bad. If autophagy is hampered, the cellular damage spreads, promoting premature aging and disease. Your body has to divert resources to digestion when you eat, so it doesn't have time for cellular cleanup. When you restrict food intake, your body has time and resources to spare, making intermittent fasting an important driver of autophagy.[29, 30]

Improved Gut Health

Your *gut* is a generic term that refers to your intestines. We used to think that the intestines were nothing more than a long tube that allowed for the digestion and absorption of food. We now know that it is a complex system that is filled with bugs! (That's a good thing, by the way.) Those bugs form a community of beneficial bacteria that are collectively referred to as your gut microbiome. In the past few decades, the health of your gut microbiome has been linked to the health of your immune system, your ability to control your weight, and the prevention of gastrointestinal conditions such as inflammatory bowel disease.[31, 32]

Your gut bacteria feed off of the fiber and scraps of undigested foods that you eat, so it's easy to see how your food choices matter when it comes to the health of your gut microbiome. But interestingly, the health of your gut may also be related to the timing of food consumption. It is thought that the bacteria in the gut microbiome experience daily rhythms, and the timing of eating may positively modulate daily changes in the diversity and abundance of gut bacteria.[33, 34] The rest that the gut experiences during a fast may also prove beneficial by reducing gut permeability, or leaky gut, a condition in which bacteria and toxins "leak" through the protective wall of the intestine and enter the bloodstream, where they can cause inflammation and disease.[34, 35]

FASTING AND MUSCLE LOSS

Even with the reassurance that your body can perform well and even thrive while fasting, you might still feel cautious about skipping a meal, thinking that the lack of food coming in will cause your body to lose muscle. This is a valid concern because muscle is important to quality of life, and carrying more muscle with you into your senior years has been linked to longevity.[39]

As discussed earlier in the chapter, when you adopt a fasting lifestyle, your body becomes metabolically flexible, meaning that it can efficiently switch between running on

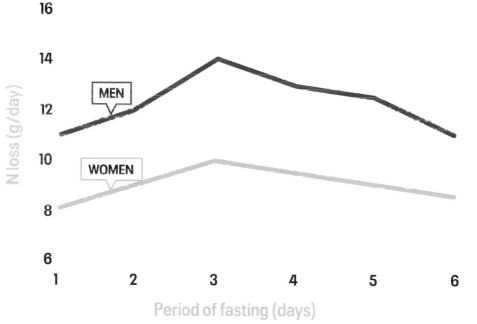

Muscle loss and fasting

Change in urea nitrogen (N) excretion in obese subjects during the first 6 days of fasting

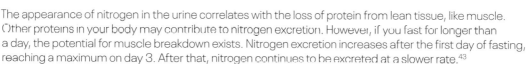

The appearance of nitrogen in the urine correlates with the loss of protein from lean tissue, like muscle. Other proteins in your body may contribute to nitrogen excretion. However, if you fast for longer than a day, the potential for muscle breakdown exists. Nitrogen excretion increases after the first day of fasting, reaching a maximum on day 3. After that, nitrogen continues to be excreted at a slower rate.[43]

glucose, fatty acids, ketones, or amino acids. Amino acids, the building blocks of muscle, are not a preferred fuel source, but they can be burned if necessary. Fortunately, your body works to conserve protein when there is no food coming in, likely because protein is an expensive fuel. Protein is a needed building block for countless structures in your body, from muscle fibers, to enzymes, to hormones. Burning protein for fuel would be like burning money to heat your home. You'd stay warm for a little while, but you'd lose out in the long run.

A study published in *Nutrition Reviews* in 2015 looked at the effects of intermittent fasting on body composition by reviewing many previously published studies to learn more about the effects of fasting on muscle. The researchers noticed that fasting could result in the presence of more *urea nitrogen,* which is a waste product that is created when the body breaks down proteins like the ones that make up muscle. However, that increase does not show up until a person has been fasting for consecutive days; the brief fast you perform by skipping a meal and other shorter fasts lasting less than a day will not appreciably break down your muscles for energy.[40]

There is evidence that prolonged fasting can result in some muscle breakdown, but exactly when this occurs is not clear. One study that was reviewed showed that lean, healthy men did not experience metabolic protein changes when performing short-term alternate-day fasting (alternating between 20 hours of fasting and 28 hours of feeding). Another study showed that evidence of muscle breakdown increased at 60 hours.[40]

What happens in your body during a day of fasting?

Let's recap all of the amazing things happening inside your body during a day of fasting! When you fast, your body uses stored energy to run your metabolism, repair tissues, and clean up damaged cells and debris. Here's an overview of the biological processes.

4-6 hours

- **Your stomach empties.**

- **Ghrelin increases.** This hunger hormone is produced by your empty stomach, creating the first subtle wave of hunger. After that initial wave, ghrelin decreases, and hunger is reduced. It will continue to rise and fall throughout your fast.

6-12 hours

- **Your digestive system goes to rest.** Nutrients from your last meal have been absorbed into your bloodstream, where insulin moved them to your cells for storage. With insulin's job completed, secretions diminish.

- **Your body runs on stored glucose.** With no energy coming in, your liver maintains a stable blood sugar level by breaking down glycogen (stored glucose).

- **Your body shifts from running on sugar to running on fat.** With relatively little energy stored in glycogen, reserves quickly diminish, setting the stage for fat burning.

So, what is the length of time that you can fast without concern of muscle loss? In the chart on page 47, we see that muscle may be breaking down as early as the first full day of fasting, as shown by the rise in urea nitrogen that occurs at 24 hours. As the fast continues, nitrogen excretion rises until day 3, at which time it slows but does not stop. This slowing of the rate may indicate an attempt by the body to conserve muscle during prolonged fasts.[41, 42]

It's hard to predict the exact tipping point when a fast will begin to result in muscle loss. However, we do know that when individuals (who are adequately nourished) fast for fewer than 24 hours or alternate between fasting and feasting days, they don't lose an appreciable amount of muscle.[24] After a day of fasting, muscle breakdown may begin.

The muscle-sparing effect seen in short-term fasts is just one example of the amazing adaptability of the human body. You live in a machine that never stops. Even when you sleep, your body is generating energy that it pulls from its natural reserves of glycogen and fat, or your liver makes new energy from nutrients that are available. When you wake, your body continues to need energy. You can provide that energy by eating breakfast, or you can let your body continue to do its thing, pulling energy from its reserves. This is the beauty of intermittent fasting!

12–24 hours

- **Your body runs on stored fat.** Adipose tissue releases free fatty acids that can be used for energy by tissues like the liver, kidneys, and muscles.

- **Ketones are produced by the liver to fuel your brain.** The brain runs well on ketones, but not on free fatty acids. Your liver converts some fatty acids to ketones to keep you mentally sharp.

- **Autophagy begins.** With the chore of digestion past, resources are diverted toward cleanup processes like autophagy, which removes damaged cells and debris.

- **Inflammation decreases throughout the body.** Levels of oxidative stress and inflammation are reduced in response to fasting.

- **The secretion of metabolic hormones increases.** Growth hormone and norepinephrine rise, supporting your metabolism as you fast.

Beyond 24 hours

- **Blood sugar and insulin levels remain low.** Extended periods of fasting may be used with a health-care provider's guidance to treat blood sugar disorders and further reduce disease-causing inflammation in your body.

- **Urea nitrogen excretion starts to rise.** Urea nitrogen is a waste product that is produced from the breakdown of protein. The increase in excretion could indicate the start of muscle loss.

4

DIFFERENT APPROACHES TO FASTING

What lies ahead

There are three main ways to fast:

- **Time-restricted eating (TRE):** With this method, you eat every day, but you consume all of your calories within a set number of hours. Popular TRE strategies include 12:12, 16:8, 20:4, and one-meal-a-day (OMAD).

- **Alternate-day fasting:** As the name implies, this method involves alternating between fasting and nonfasting days. Modified versions allow for the consumption of 20 to 25 percent of your energy needs (approximately 500–600 calories) on fasting days.

- **Extended (prolonged) fasting:** Fasts that last longer than 24 hours are classified as extended or prolonged fasts.

eople have been fasting for
religious or healing purposes
for millennia. So fasting in and
of itself is nothing new. What is new
is using fasting as a way to lose
weight and gain health in our
modern world of abundance. This
chapter will introduce you to
different ways to fast so you can
compare methods and consider
their pros and cons.

TIME-RESTRICTED EATING VS. INTERMITTENT FASTING

Before we jump into the different approaches,
it's beneficial to clarify some terminology,
specifically the difference between time-
restricted eating and intermittent fasting.
The term *time-restricted eating* (or *feeding*)
was coined by researcher Dr. Satchin Panda
to designate a way of fasting that aligns
with a body's natural circadian rhythm
without calorie restriction. *Intermittent
fasting* is a broad term that encompasses
multiple eating patterns in which there are
fasting and nonfasting periods that may
or may not consider calories. Outside of
the research world, the difference comes
down to semantics, and the terms are used
interchangeably. For the purposes of this
book, I am using the term *time-restricted
eating* (TRE) to describe methods of fasting
that allow you to eat every day within
a shortened eating window. The term
intermittent fasting is used as an umbrella
term to describe single- or multiple-day
eating and fasting patterns.

GETTING STARTED

If you've never fasted before, you should start
out with a TRE pattern such as 12:12 or 16:8.
After a few days of testing the waters, you'll
have an idea about how to wait out hunger
pangs to stay on track.

Intermittent fasting is flexible, so consider
your schedule and the needs of your family
members or a job; make the fasting pattern
work for you! You'll quickly learn how to
adapt the patterns to how you're feeling—
there is no right or wrong way to go about it.
See the next chapter for advice on making
your goals and choosing a fasting schedule.

As you're reading through each of the
patterns in this chapter, you may find it
motivating to cross-reference the art at
the bottom of pages 48 and 49. It's exciting
to understand the hour-by-hour benefits
you will be giving your body!

With that understanding in mind, let's take a
look at exactly how to fast, starting with the
easiest method—12:12 fasting.

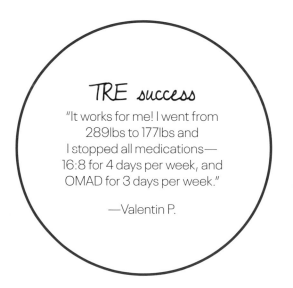

TRE success

"It works for me! I went from
289lbs to 177lbs and
I stopped all medications—
16:8 for 4 days per week, and
OMAD for 3 days per week."

—Valentin P.

Intermittent fasting schedules

You've probably heard the buzzwords and have some idea of the types of fasting available to you. Here is a comparison of the primary types so you can see your options.

Time-restricted eating patterns split your **day** between periods of eating and fasting														
12:12 fasting	Eat	Fast	Eat	Fast	Eat	Fast	Eat	Fast	Eat	Fast	Eat	Fast	Eat	Fast
16:8 fasting	Eat	Fast	Eat	Fast	Eat	Fast	Eat	Fast	Eat	Fast	Eat	Fast	Eat	Fast
20:4 fasting	Eat	Fast	Eat	Fast	Eat	Fast	Eat	Fast	Eat	Fast	Eat	Fast	Eat	Fast
OMAD	Fast		Fast		Fast		Fast		Fast		Fast		Fast	
	DAY 1		DAY 2		DAY 3		DAY 4		DAY 5		DAY 6		DAY 7	

Alternate day fasting (ADF) schedules split your **week** between periods of eating and fasting							
Full ADF	Eat normally	Fast	Eat normally	Fast	Eat normally	Fast	Eat normally
Modified ADF	Eat normally	Eat 500 calories	Eat normally	Eat 500 calories	Eat normally	Eat 500 calories	Eat normally
The 5:2 Diet	Eat normally	Eat 500–600 calories	Eat normally	Eat normally	Eat 500–600 calories	Eat normally	Eat normally
	DAY 1	DAY 2	DAY 3	DAY 4	DAY 5	DAY 6	DAY 7

Extended fasting schedules last **more than 24 hours** and are performed periodically throughout the year							
Extended fast	Eat normally	Fast	Fast	Fast	Eat normally	Eat normally	Eat normally
	DAY 1	DAY 2	DAY 3	DAY 4	DAY 5	DAY 6	DAY 7

12:12 FASTING

This entry-level fasting method is a great place to start. Think of it as an overnight fast like you might do when preparing for a blood test. If your doctor schedules a blood test for the next morning, he or she may ask you to stop eating after dinner and not resume eating until after your test the next morning. Performing a 12-hour fast is no more complicated than that.

How to Do It

A 12:12 fast splits your day in half. You'll consume all of your daily calories within a 12-hour eating window and fast for the other 12 hours of the day. This method is all about getting comfortable with fasting. You can read about IF and think it sounds great, but when it comes time to try it, fears rush in:

- Will I be hungry?
- Will I feel sick?
- Will fasting cause me to overeat in the remaining hours of the day?

12:12 fasting

A 12-hour fast is easiest to do if you include the hours you sleep in the fasting window. Eat as many meals as you'd like during your eating window. Here is a sample of how you could plan your day.

	DAY 1	DAY 2	DAY 3	DAY 4	DAY 5	DAY 6	DAY 7
Midnight – 4am	Fast	Fast	Fast	Fast	Fast	Fast	Fast
8am – Noon	First meal at 7am	First meal at 7am	First meal at 7am	First meal at 7am	First meal at 7am	First meal at 7am	First meal at 7am
4pm	Last meal by 7pm	Last meal by 7pm	Last meal by 7 pm	Last meal by 7pm	Last meal by 7pm	Last meal by 7pm	Last meal by 7pm
8pm – Midnight	Fast	Fast	Fast	Fast	Fast	Fast	Fast

It is normal to feel some uncertainty when you begin intermittent fasting. Starting with a 12:12 fast will calm your fears and build your confidence.

Fasting is easiest to do if you include the hours that you sleep. To get started, have dinner as you normally would. There's no need to eat an extra serving at dinner to tide you over; you'll be fine. Note the time you stopped eating—that time is the start of your fast. Feel free to have some water or tea in the evening hours before you go to bed, but don't consume food or caloric drinks. (If you're having trouble avoiding late-night snacking, try brushing and flossing your teeth. Your mouth will feel fresh and clean, which will help curb cravings and make you think twice before dirtying it with more food.) When 12 hours have passed, you can break your fast with your normal breakfast. You did it! The only thing left to do is note how you feel. I'm going to bet that you feel good and have a feeling of optimism that you can do this!

Pros: You can eat three or more meals as you normally would during the day as long as you restrict the window during which you consume calories to 12 hours.

Cons: This relatively short period without food may help stabilize blood sugar and maintain weight, but the full weight loss and health benefits of intermittent fasting will not be realized.

Who is it right for? If you are just getting started and feeling apprehensive about how you'll feel while fasting, this method is right for you.

Extra tip: When you feel comfortable with 12-hour fasting, take the next step by

increasing your fasting period to 14 hours. For example, finish dinner by 7pm and postpone breakfast until 9am. Consistent adherence to a 10-hour eating window has been shown to result in a reduction of weight and improved energy and sleep.[1]

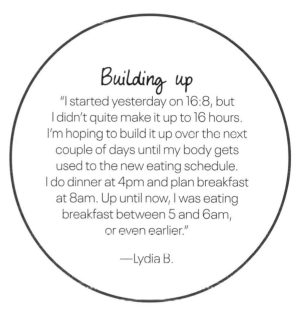

Building up

"I started yesterday on 16:8, but I didn't quite make it up to 16 hours. I'm hoping to build it up over the next couple of days until my body gets used to the new eating schedule. I do dinner at 4pm and plan breakfast at 8am. Up until now, I was eating breakfast between 5 and 6am, or even earlier."

—Lydia B.

16:8 FASTING

This is when the magic starts happening! With 16 hours of fasting behind you, your blood sugar and insulin levels are low, some of the stored glucose (glycogen) has been depleted, and your body is looking for fuel. Fortunately, your adipose (fat) tissue has plenty of energy to give. This period without food also gives your body time off from the energy-demanding job of digesting food, which frees up the resources needed for healing and repair.

16:8 fasting

Fasting from after dinner to lunch the next day is a common way to perform a 16:8 fast. Here is a sample of how you could plan your day. You could eat two or three meals during your eating window.

	DAY 1	DAY 2	DAY 3	DAY 4	DAY 5	DAY 6	DAY 7
Midnight – 4am – 8am	Fast	Fast	Fast	Fast	Fast	Fast	Fast
Noon – 4pm	First meal at 11am / Last meal by 7pm	First meal at 11am / Last meal by 7pm	First meal at 11am / Last meal by 7pm	First meal at 11am / Last meal by 7pm	First meal at 11am / Last meal by 7pm	First meal at 11am / Last meal by 7pm	First meal at 11am / Last meal by 7pm
8pm – Midnight	Fast	Fast	Fast	Fast	Fast	Fast	Fast

How to Do It

Although you can choose any 16 hours to fast, many people find that finishing their eating window with dinner and then skipping breakfast the next day is the easiest way to complete a 16:8 fast.

If you intend to skip breakfast, it's helpful to think about how you'll handle your morning hours. Coffee is okay to consume, as is tea or water. A bit of cream in your coffee or tea can help quiet hunger and add to the enjoyment of your morning, but watch out for "calorie creep." Cream is mainly fat. Because dietary fat does not raise your blood sugar or insulin levels, it doesn't block fat burning. However, the fat calories from the cream provide your body with an easily accessible energy source, causing your body to step away from burning body fat until the calories are used up. If you're drinking three cups of coffee in the morning and adding cream to each cup, your calories are creeping up to a level that matches your body's energy needs. Remember that fasting is effective for weight loss because it robs your body of easy energy, forcing it to tap into harder-to-access body fat. It is also worth noting that consuming any calories during your fast may interrupt autophagy or other healing processes, so if you are looking to use fasting for health benefits as well as weight loss, then you will be happiest with your results if you skip the add-ins and drink your coffee or tea black.

Pros: 16:8 fasting meets the three E's (easy to do, enjoyable, and effective). Skipping breakfast is *easy* for many people because hunger is naturally lower in the morning, and the busyness associated with this time of day helps keep their minds off of eating. Dinner can be *enjoyed* with the family. And fasting for 16 hours is *effective* for health and weight loss.

Cons: Fasting after dinner until lunch the next day requires you to avoid after-dinner drinks and snacks, and you'll need to reduce or eliminate coffee creamer. These lifestyle adjustments can be challenging.

Who is it right for? If you naturally feel less hungry in the morning, you'll find it easy to skip breakfast and complete a 16-hour fast. If you do well with a structured routine, you will enjoy the predictability of this method of fasting.

Extra tip: For the best results, eat two or three meals during your eating window. Grazing throughout the entire 8-hour window continually bumps up your blood sugar and insulin level, which can block the release of fat from your fat cells.

Fast fact: use a "fat fast" to combat hunger

A **fat fast** is not an official form of intermittent fasting, but it is something you might find helpful if you struggle with getting started due to hunger. With a fat fast, you can consume pure fat foods during your fasting window. For instance, you could add cream, MCT oil, butter, or other fats to your coffee until your hunger abates. If hunger continues, high-fat foods like eggs, avocados, cheese, or olives could be added in small amounts until you feel in control.

Dietary fat is hunger satiating and does not spike blood sugar or insulin, allowing your body to stay in a fat-burning state. If you are struggling with hunger, don't throw in the towel! Use a fat fast as a crutch until you feel comfortable with fasting and then wean yourself off the fats to improve your results.

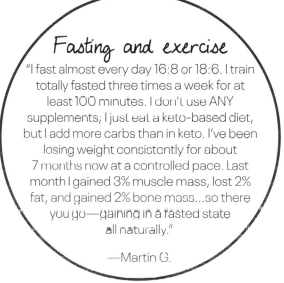

Fasting and exercise

"I fast almost every day 16:8 or 18:6. I train totally fasted three times a week for at least 100 minutes. I don't use ANY supplements; I just eat a keto-based diet, but I add more carbs than in keto. I've been losing weight consistently for about 7 months now at a controlled pace. Last month I gained 3% muscle mass, lost 2% fat, and gained 2% bone mass...so there you go—gaining in a fasted state all naturally."

—Martin G.

20:4 FASTING (A.K.A. THE WARRIOR DIET)

It's questionable if the benefits derived from a 20-hour fast are substantially superior to those obtained from a 16-hour fast. However, 20:4 fasting has captured the interest of many individuals who are looking to step up their progress. Fitness expert Ori Hofmekler popularized this fasting schedule.

20:4 fasting

To practice this strategy, consume all of your day's calories within 4 hours. Here is a sample of how you could plan your day, eating two meals or a meal and a snack.

	DAY 1	DAY 2	DAY 3	DAY 4	DAY 5	DAY 6	DAY 7
Midnight – Noon	Fast	Fast	Fast	Fast	Fast	Fast	Fast
Noon – 8pm	First meal at 2pm / Last meal by 6pm	First meal at 2pm / Last meal by 6pm	First meal at 2pm / Last meal by 6pm	First meal at 2pm / Last meal by 6pm	First meal at 2pm / Last meal by 6pm	First meal at 2pm / Last meal by 6pm	First meal at 2pm / Last meal by 6pm
8pm – Midnight	Fast	Fast	Fast	Fast	Fast	Fast	Fast

Hofmekler nicknamed the fast the Warrior Diet because he patterned it after ancient warrior tribes who would eat small amounts of whole, unprocessed foods during the day and one large meal in the evening.

How to Do It

The original Warrior Diet specified a particular eating style that emphasized consuming a hearty, drawn-out evening meal filled with plenty of protein, unprocessed carbohydrates, and healthy fats. Today, many people look at fasting for 20 hours as a way to push their bodies to a higher level of fat burning and cellular repair, although there have been few studies performed to support these benefits.[2]

To perform a 20:4 fast, you'll want to consume all your daily calories within a 4-hour eating window. Those calories could be consumed in any way that fits your lifestyle, but one strategy would be to have two meals between 2pm and 6pm.

There's something compelling about fasting for 20 hours of a 24-hour day, but this method is not for everyone. The original Warrior Diet stressed the importance of consuming whole, unprocessed foods during the eating window. It's easy to see how ancient warriors could have benefited from this strategy because clean, nutrient-dense foods were the only foods available. Today, we live in a world filled with calorie-dense, nutrient-poor foods. Without careful planning, it could be easy to binge on fast foods and processed snacks, decreasing the health value of this strategy. For that reason, you may want to look at more extensive fasts like this one as an occasional strategy that is intended to temporarily ramp up your progress or break you out of a weight-loss plateau.

Pros: Those with a stubborn metabolism may find that 20 hours of fasting is what their body needs to lose weight. It could also be argued that the additional hours of low blood sugar and insulin may benefit those with blood sugar disorders.

Cons: If you jump into this method too quickly, you may experience hunger and cravings that lead to binge eating. You'll be happiest with your experience if you approach a 20:4 fast as an intermediate skill level to practice after you've become comfortable with 16:8 fasting.

Who is it right for? If you have trouble losing weight or your weight loss has plateaued, you may find that extending your fasting window to 20 hours does the trick.

Extra tip: Stop eating at least 3 hours before bed. When food is in your system, blood flow is directed to your digestive tract. This central blood flow raises your core body temperature, which can interfere with sleep. Also, your cells become less sensitive to insulin as the evening progresses, so eating a meal close to bedtime causes blood glucose levels to remain elevated overnight.[2]

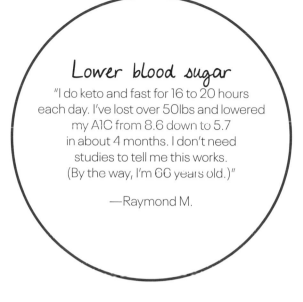

Lower blood sugar

"I do keto and fast for 16 to 20 hours each day. I've lost over 50lbs and lowered my A1C from 8.6 down to 5.7 in about 4 months. I don't need studies to tell me this works. (By the way, I'm 66 years old.)"

—Raymond M.

OMAD (ONE MEAL A DAY)

OMAD is an acronym that stands for "one meal a day." That meal is generally consumed over the course of an hour, so OMAD can also be thought of as a 23 hour fast, or 23:1 fasting. This approach is the most extreme form of time-restricted eating.

How to Do It

Eating one time per day is an easy concept to grasp. The meal can last for 1 hour and can be thought of as a large meal without calorie or macronutrient limits. That said, gorging on processed, refined carbs is not encouraged. However, the reality is that when eating healthy, whole foods, it is challenging to take in sufficient calories to meet your body's needs. This outcome can be looked at in a positive or negative light. The positive impact is that limiting food intake to one meal per day naturally creates a caloric deficit that encourages weight loss. However, stringing too many low-calorie days together tends to lower your resting metabolic rate, which makes long-term weight control difficult. This negative outcome was famously demonstrated in a study done on participants of *The Biggest Loser* who experienced metabolic consequences that persisted for years after the show ended. During the competition, contestants drastically decreased their calorie intake and increased their calorie expenditure through exercise. The chronic caloric deficit resulted in rapid weight loss. Unfortunately, it also caused their metabolisms to drop to a level that was more in line with their calorie restriction.[3]

In other words, their bodies adapted to the new low level of calories by burning fewer calories, making it very easy to regain the weight that they had lost.

Research studies on time-restricted eating rarely capture a true one-meal-a-day pattern that involves consuming all calories within a 1-hour eating window, so with that limited research, we are left to speculate about the benefits and risks. With the limited research and concerns about chronic calorie restriction, eating one meal a day may best be looked as a way to throw your metabolism a curveball, which keeps it from becoming stagnant, rather than an everyday practice.

OMAD (One Meal a Day)

OMAD condenses your eating window to 1 hour per day, making it the most extreme TRE pattern. You could choose to eat your one meal any time of the day.

	DAY 1	DAY 2	DAY 3	DAY 4	DAY 5	DAY 6	DAY 7
Midnight 4am 8am Noon	Fast	Fast	Fast	Fast	Fast	Fast	Fast
4pm	1 meal in 1 hour	1 meal in 1 hour	1 meal in 1 hour	1 meal in 1 hour	1 meal in 1 hour	1 meal in 1 hour	1 meal in 1 hour
8pm Midnight	Fast	Fast	Fast	Fast	Fast	Fast	Fast

Pros: Throwing an OMAD fast into your weekly routine may help you to break a weight-loss plateau. If you are traveling or have a particularly busy day, OMAD simplifies life by reducing the time needed for food preparation and eating.

Cons: Narrowing your eating window to 1 hour a day makes it challenging to get all of the nutrients and calories needed to prevent a slowing of your metabolism. If you perform this method regularly, you'll be happiest with your results if you closely monitor your body fat percentage to make sure that you are losing fat, not muscle.

Who is it right for? If you're stuck at a weight-loss plateau, looking for a challenge, or traveling with limited time to eat, OMAD is worthwhile.

Extra tip: Many people feel good when they eat one meal a day, but it's not for everyone. Although hunger and light fatigue are expected and acceptable consequences of OMAD, you should stop your fast if you are feeling extremely fatigued, light-headed, nauseated, or unusually unwell in any way.

Feeling good in her skin

"I do OMAD. All my bloating is gone, my pants are significantly looser, and I feel better. The scale is my kryptonite, so I am going by how I look and feel through this, as my goal is just to get healthier and feel better about myself. I am very hopeful with this, and it's easy for me because I was a breakfast skipper anyway. Now I skip lunch too, so it's not a big jump."

—Maggie M.

ALTERNATE-DAY FASTING

Alternate-day fasts, as you would expect, are performed by alternating between fasting and nonfasting days. There are two versions that I will refer to as *full* and *modified*. A full alternate-day fast requires you to completely abstain from caloric food and drink every other day. The modified method allows you to consume about 500 calories on your fasting days.

How to Do It

Performing a full alternate-day fast means that you consume no calories on your fasting days. For instance, you could finish eating dinner on Monday, avoid food on Tuesday, and then resume eating on Wednesday. During the fasting period, you can consume noncaloric drinks, like water, coffee, and tea. During the eating window, eat to your satisfaction level.

Dr. Krista Varady is one of the leading researchers on alternate-day fasting. She found that modifying the fasting days by allowing the consumption of 20 to 25 percent of your body's energy needs (typically simplified to 500 calories) increases adherence without sacrificing the health and weight-loss benefits. Your 500-calorie allotment on fasting days can be consumed as one meal or a small meal and snacks. The nonfasting days are looked at as feasting days, meaning you can consume food until your hunger is satisfied.

With both versions, there are no limitations on calorie intake or food choices on your nonfasting days. I understand the appeal of this concept, but you might be concerned that this on-again, off-again style of eating could lead to binge eating. Although studies show that participants who performed alternate-day fasts tended to eat more than normal on nonfasting days, the amount that they consumed was not enough to overcome the reduction of calories from fasting days.[4, 5] So the weight loss seen with consistent alternate-day fasting is due, in part, to the fact that calorie intake is naturally decreased over time.

Pros: Alternate-day fasting is one of the most studied methods of fasting, with both versions showing positive health and weight-loss benefits.[6, 7] Many people find that they have an easier time sticking with an alternate-day fasting routine than to more traditional diets that restrict calories daily.[4, 5]

Cons: It's possible that completely going without food for more than a day, as done with the full version, may cause a loss of muscle mass.[8] (Fortunately, the modified version seems to protect against the loss of muscle.[7]) Both versions require discipline,

Alternate-day fasting

Fasting days can be full fasts with no calorie intake or modified fasts that allow 500 calories. Here is a sample of how you could plan your week.

DAY 1	DAY 2	DAY 3	DAY 4	DAY 5	DAY 6	DAY 7
Eat normally	Full-day fast OR Eat 500 calories	Eat normally	Full-day fast OR Eat 500 calories	Eat normally	Full-day fast OR Eat 500 calories	Eat normally

and hunger may become an issue on fasting days. Please note that the research that has been done on this and other forms of alternate-day fasting took place over many weeks or months, so consistency may be needed to realize full benefits.

Who is it right for? Alternate-day fasting may be the push that some people are looking for to break a weight-loss plateau or coax a stubborn metabolism to burn fat. A modified fast will appeal to those who want to accelerate their results but take comfort in knowing that they can eat something on fasting days and eat to their satisfaction level the next day.

Extra tip: You have the freedom to eat whatever you want every other day. There is no doubt that this idea captures the imagination and conjures up an image of an endless smorgasbord of treats. However, if you are looking at these methods of fasting as a way to eat with abandon, you could suffer health consequences and make your fasting experience less enjoyable. Regular consumption of fast foods and processed snacks has little health value and can lead to unstable blood sugar levels that drive cravings. If alternate-day fasting is something that interests you, you'll be happiest with your health and weight-loss results if you choose whole, unprocessed foods.

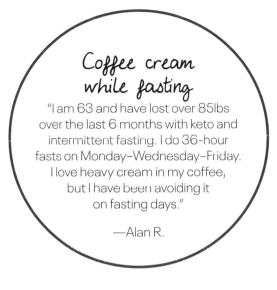

Coffee cream while fasting

"I am 63 and have lost over 85lbs over the last 6 months with keto and intermittent fasting. I do 36-hour fasts on Monday–Wednesday–Friday. I love heavy cream in my coffee, but I have been avoiding it on fasting days."

—Alan R.

THE 5:2 DIET

Fast for 2 days of the week—that is the basic concept behind the 5:2 diet. This spin on alternate-day fasting was popularized by Dr. Michael Mosley and is also known as The Fast Diet. The protocol involves limiting your calories for 2 days of the week and eating as you normally would for 5 days.

How to Do It

When following this protocol, the days you choose to fast are up to you, but they should not be consecutive days. So you could fast on Monday and Thursday, but you would not want to fast on Monday and Tuesday. Like the modified version of alternate-day fasting, you are allowed to consume 500 calories on your fasting days with some sources saying that men could consume 600 calories. Those fasting-day calories can be consumed in a single meal or spread out into smaller meals.

The 5:2 diet

This twist on alternate-day fasting has you perform a modified fast 2 days of the week. Here is a sample of how you could plan your week. Do not plan your fasting days on consecutive days.

DAY 1	DAY 2	DAY 3	DAY 4	DAY 5	DAY 6	DAY 7
Eat normally	Eat 500–600 calories	Eat normally	Eat normally	Eat 500–600 calories	Eat normally	Eat normally

Like the other forms of alternate-day fasting, the 5:2 diet is effective for weight loss. This benefit might be because calories are naturally reduced for the week. One 6-month study compared two groups of overweight women. One group was placed on a traditional low-calorie diet that cut their daily caloric intake by 25 percent. The other group followed a 5:2 diet routine by dramatically restricting their calories on 2 days of the week and then eating normally on the other 5 days. Analysis at the end of the study showed that the two groups took in about the same level of calories and macronutrients, despite their different patterns of eating.[9] This result again seems to indicate that alternate-day fasting does not cause binge eating as some might expect.

Pros: Unlike other forms of alternate-day fasting, the 5:2 model limits calories on just 2 days of the week rather than every other day. Although effort is still required, this method is the least restrictive and, therefore, the easier entry point for those interested in alternate-day fasting.

Cons: As with any extreme calorie restriction, you may get side effects like irritability, hunger, or difficulty sleeping. Plus, 5 days of "normal" eating could be a slippery slope for some people in terms of food choices. It is human nature to want to reward yourself after doing hard work, which could translate into eating more junk food than you normally would on your nonfasting days.

Who is it right for? Whether you're new to fasting or experienced and looking for ways to vary your routine, 5:2 fasting is worth a look. Unlike the built-in structure of other alternate-day fasting routines, the 5:2 diet allows you to pick which days you fast. The freedom to schedule your low-calorie days makes this strategy appealing to those with busy social calendars.

Extra tip: Despite a 500-calorie allowance on fasting days, hunger is a reality for most people who practice this type of fast. However, your level of hunger may diminish the longer you follow the protocol. One study found that participants experienced an increase in hunger during their first week of fasting, but their hunger scores decreased after week 2 and remained low throughout the remainder of the study.[5]

Planning for 5:2 dieters

"I've done IF for over 2 years, usually OMAD on work days. I've recently dabbled in 5:2 and full ADF to break through weight loss plateaus, and I've quite enjoyed it. It's very easy to follow (especially if you plan out your day, your work schedule, etc.). Some might need that 500 calories to get through the fasting days at first, but for me, it's easier to have no calories and just drink sparkling water and coffee or tea."

—Tony O.

EXTENDED FASTING

The definition of an extended or prolonged fast varies from one source to the next. I define it as a fast lasting longer than a day. There are potential benefits with long-term fasting, such as increased weight loss, enhanced autophagy, and consistently stable blood sugar and insulin levels, but there are also risks. The risks include, but are not limited to, the loss of muscle and a drop in metabolism. If you are considering extending your fasting period longer than a day, you'll want to weigh the risks and benefits and consult your doctor before starting.

How to Do It

Because extended fasts last longer than 1 day, they can easily include 1 or more nights of sleep, making them 36, 48, or more hours long.

- **36-hour fast:** To perform this fast, you could stop eating at 7pm on day 1, skip all meals on day 2, and then resume eating at 7am on day 3.

- **48-hour fast:** To perform this fast, you could stop eating at 7pm on day 1, skip all meals on day 2, and then resume eating at 7pm on day 3.

- **Multiple-day fasts:** These fasts include multiple, consecutive days without caloric intake. There is no set protocol for how long to fast, but 3 to 7 days is a typical range.

Except for a 36-hour fast, which mimics the full alternate-day fast you learned about earlier, extended fasts are typically spaced out and performed periodically (i.e., once or twice a month) as opposed to weekly.

To perform a true extended fast, you consume nothing but water. However, noncaloric drinks such as unsweetened coffee, tea, or carbonated waters (e.g., sparkling water or club soda) can help you get through the fast and may have health benefits. There is some evidence from animal research that consuming coffee during a fast enhances autophagy.[10, 11] Certain carbonated waters contain salt and other necessary minerals that you can lose during prolonged fasts.

When you go without food for a few days, your digestive system goes through a long period of rest. You will feel your best if you gently reintroduce food at the end of your fast. I will talk more about what to consume when breaking a fast in future chapters, but for now think of low-calorie liquid foods such as bone broth. If your fast lasted for a week or longer or you enter an extended fast undernourished, the reintroduction of food must be approached with added caution to avoid a potentially life-threatening condition known as *refeeding syndrome*.[12] Although this condition is rare, when it happens, it creates a dangerous fluctuation in the fluid, vitamin, and mineral balances in the body, which reemphasizes the need for medical supervision when doing an extended fast.

Pros: When properly supervised by a medical professional, extended fasts may benefit a person with health conditions related to

Extended fasting

Extended fasts last longer than one day and are best done under medical supervision.

DAY 1	DAY 2	DAY 3	DAY 4	DAY 5	DAY 6	DAY 7
Eat normally	Fast	Fast	Fast	Eat normally	Eat normally	Eat normally

obesity. The extended fasting period keeps insulin levels low, which may be what is needed to overcome blood sugar disorders.

Cons: You will be going without food for consecutive days, which will be disruptive to family dinners and social situations. Extended fasts require supervision, especially if you are taking medications that are affected by your diet. For instance, if you are taking insulin for diabetes but not eating, your medication will need to be adjusted from day 1 of the fast. Other medications may need to be taken with food to improve absorption or avoid stomach upset.

Who is it right for? Extended fasts are most advantageous for those under medical supervision for conditions like obesity, diabetes, heart disease, and cancer.

Extra tip: Exercise is not forbidden during an extended fast, but intense exercise may prove to be difficult, and your performance can suffer. Trying to push your body to lose weight by putting it through extreme exercise could backfire, resulting in the breakdown of muscle or increased hunger

TAKING YOUR NEXT STEP

From 12-hour overnight fasts to prolonged fasts that last for multiple days, there are many fasting methods to choose from. As we moved through this chapter, you likely found yourself drawn to certain strategies, but which one is right for you? In the next chapter, we'll take your lifestyle, work schedule, and goals into consideration to determine your best path into the world of intermittent fasting. It's time to jump in!

Breaking through a plateau

"I was stuck using intermittent fasting after losing 50lbs. I decided to do a 36-hour fast and BAM—that moved the scale. Our bodies truly adapt, don't they? So until I hit another plateau, I will stay with my 16:8 intermittent fasting. It suits my life, and I'll be happy with losing a pound a week doing this."

—Eileen V.

5

MAKING YOUR GOAL + DECIDING ON A FASTING METHOD

What lies ahead

- **We are all unique!** You can choose a fasting schedule that fits you and your lifestyle.

- **Fasting routines can be fine-tuned to meet your goals and needs.** Whether you want to build muscle, lose weight, rejuvenate your health, or stay healthy amid a hectic life, there's a fasting method to help.

Fasting is a wonderful tool for getting your health and weight on track. With a bit of experimentation, you'll find what works best for you. Go into fasting with the mindset that your body is your friend and ally. If you help your friend, your friend will help you. When you give your body time off from the chore of digesting food, you help it by freeing up energy and resources to do other things. In return, your body gives you better health and weight control.

SETTING YOUR GOAL

Have you given thought to what you'd like to accomplish through IF? Is weight loss your primary focus? Are you looking to regain an aspect of your health that has been lost or enhance your health as you age? Would you like more energy or improved mental clarity?

When it comes to IF, there is no one-size-fits-all approach. The method that feels right to you will depend on many factors; some are within your control, including your enthusiasm level and determination to see results, and others are not. Factors outside of your control include your gender, age, existing metabolic issues, family needs, and work schedule. All of these factors play into choosing the right approach for you as a unique individual. For instance, young adults who are interested in preserving muscle mass while getting lean may find timing their workouts with their fasting schedule is best. A woman of reproductive years will benefit from a less-extreme form of fasting to avoid changes in her menstrual cycle. Those who have slower-performing metabolisms due to advanced age, hormonal issues, or years of being overweight and eating a nutrient-poor diet may find that a strong adherence to daily fasting is needed to realize results. Those with active family lives and demanding work schedules will require a more flexible and fluid fasting schedule.

Regardless of your goal and the factors that make your life unique, fasting is a valuable tool in your toolbox. But let's address the elephant you might see standing in the room—fear. What if you don't think you can fast? I assure you that you are not alone in your uneasiness. It's common to feel a measure of anxiety at this stage in the game. However, I also assure you that your fears will melt away with action. Let me help you get started and then set you free with some individual strategies for your unique life.

Starting slow

"I started with the 12:12 schedule because initially going without food for that long was a challenge. I was a nighttime nibbler. I began with not eating 3 hours before bed— just that was an accomplishment. As I continued, I can now do 16:8 very easily, which I never thought I could."

—Lorna H.

A GENERAL GAME PLAN

If you're enthusiastic about getting started and in generally good health, there is nothing wrong with jumping into a longer time-restricted eating schedule, alternate-day routine, or even going a full day without food. However, keep in mind that your body will not be on board right away, which could lead to hunger, fatigue, and mentally feeling a bit off. Your body likes the routine that you have established. You wake up, go to the bathroom, shower, grab a cup of coffee, and your body is right there with you motoring along on autopilot. *Yes,* it thinks, *we have started another blissfully normal day! The next thing we'll do is eat breakfast—great, bring it on!*

Except today you have a different plan. Today, you are going to skip breakfast and put off your first meal until noon. Your body is in no danger. It has stocked up fuel for a time like this. However, this change in routine throws your body for a loop. It had already decided that this is a typical day, so it continues to run on autopilot. Because you're not playing along, it gives you a nudge by secreting ghrelin, a hunger hormone produced from your now-empty stomach. Ghrelin delivers a message to your brain, telling it that you haven't eaten in a while, so it would be good to turn up the volume on hunger. "Our person seems to have forgotten breakfast. Let's give her a reminder that it is time to eat." If you stick to your guns, you'll continue to confuse your body. It was planning on receiving fuel this morning, but with no food to process, it is forced to tap into stored energy. This is a task that it was not ready to perform, so your energy runs low and you spend the morning wrestling between cravings for a donut and the desire to curl up in a ball and take a nap. If you continue to practice IF, your body will accept your new routine. The hunger you experienced when you first started to fast may tap you on the shoulder and grab your attention, but it will soon abate naturally, and you'll be rewarded with a good level of energy and mental alertness.

A beginner's calendar

You can increase your fasting window at your own pace, but if you like structure, here's a plan you can follow:

* **Week 1:** 12 hours of fasting each day (e.g., 7pm to 7am)

* **Week 2:** 14 hours of fasting on weekdays and 12 hours through the weekend

* **Week 3:** 16 hours of fasting on the weekdays and 14 hours through the weekend

* **Week 4:** 18 hours of fasting every day of the week

If you'd like to avoid as much discomfort as possible as you transform into a fasting aficionado, start with a 12-hour fast. By declaring an end to your eating day after dinner and postponing breakfast until 12 hours have passed, your body and mind stay calm. You might experience a small twinge of hunger, but it is not going to set off craving alarms that make you feel out of control. Continue with this routine, and your body will adapt quickly, allowing you to widen your fasting window to 14 and then 16 hours without a hitch. You'll be amazed at how productive and energized you feel in the fasted state, and with signs like stable blood sugar and weight loss starting to show, you'll be able to experience for yourself the stickiness factor of fasting.

HITTING YOUR STRIDE FOR VARIOUS GOALS

Many people benefit from standard fasting strategies like 16:8 fasting and alternate-day fasting. If your main objective is to support your already-healthy lifestyle, you'll likely feel content with these fasting methods. However, if you have additional goals or an unpredictable schedule, you'll want to hone your routine. This is where the art and science of IF converge. Research is often limited in regards to using specific fasting methods to treat specific health conditions. However, we can take what we've learned from the existing research and add some common sense, clinical findings, and anecdotal evidence to fine-tune your approach. Let's work through some common goals to help you settle on your path.

Fasting Schedules for Muscle Gain

The ultimate prize for many people is to add muscle and lose fat. This favorable shift in body composition can happen with consistent effort and the right combination of fasting, exercise, and nutrition. If you think about what you are asking your body to do, you'll realize that you're asking it to tear down one structure (fat) and build another (muscle).

Which fasting schedule is right for you?

We are all different! Find a fasting schedule that works best for you and your lifestyle.

Want to build muscle?

Combine 16:8 fasting with intense exercise and adequate protein.

Are you a woman in your 20s to 40s?

Perform short-term fasts (i.e., 14 to 16 hours), or practice modified alternate-day fasting.

Do you have a stubborn metabolism?

Practice 16:8 fasting regularly and OMAD occasionally.

Do you lead a hectic life?

Skip meals when it suits your schedule.

Want to improve your overall health?

Under your doctor's supervision, practice TRE regularly, and finish eating every day by 5pm.

Surprisingly, fasting stimulates both of these processes. It encourages fat loss by reducing the calories you consume and the level of insulin in your blood. Fasting also stimulates the production of growth hormone (GH), which promotes muscle growth in adults. But as we learned on pages 47 to 49, there is a tipping point where fasting can result in muscle loss. Although the exact time frame is challenging to pinpoint, it's safe to say that fasting for longer than a day increases your potential for muscle breakdown.

The limited studies on how fasting impacts body composition tend to use 16:8 fasting as their baseline. When male and female athletes used this protocol in combination with intense weight training, they were able to maintain or build muscle mass.[1, 2] Some points of interest, however, are that study participants exercised during their eating window, and they supplemented with a whey protein drink soon after their workouts.

If your schedule requires you to work out during your fasting hours, it's hard to say if the results will be the same. I can, however, offer a personal anecdote. I tested the theory that you can build muscle in a fasted state by following a 12-week fitness program that consisted of 3 days of moderate to intense weight lifting interspersed with 3 days of high-intensity interval training (HIIT). (HIIT is a hybrid form of aerobic exercise that involves continually altering the speed and intensity of your workout.) I worked out every morning on an empty stomach and was able to build 4 pounds of muscle. Not bad for a 52-year-old lady! I did not supplement with whey protein as the study participants did, but I took creatine, a muscle-supporting supplement, before my workouts, and L-carnitine, a fat-burning supplement,

immediately after my workouts. Did these supplements break my fast? It is possible they did. However, I feel that they helped me reach my goal of adding muscle and reducing fat, so in my opinion, the benefits outweighed the temporary break in my fast.

Get Lean
by doing aerobic workouts in a fasted state

Duration of Fast	Repeat Fast
16 Hrs	Daily ▾

Start	Monday ▾	7:00pm
End	Tuesday ▾	11:00am

Aerobic exercise in a fasted state improves fat burning, glucose uptake by your muscles, and insulin sensitivity.

Nutritional considerations: Protein is needed for the support of your muscles. Unlike carbs and fat, protein is not tucked away in storage sites waiting for a need to arise. So for muscle to build, it is important that you consume enough protein to meet your body's needs. How much protein is needed during training is a debated topic and will depend on the intensity of your workouts. In the next chapter, you'll learn that consuming 15 to 25 percent of your total calories as protein is sufficient for most people. If you are exercising intensely, you'll be happiest with your results if you stay at the upper end of that range or higher. You can achieve that level through high-protein foods or supplement with protein-rich products like whey protein or branched-chain amino acids (BCAAs).

Weekly training schedule for muscle growth

Practice 16:8 fasting every day. Vary your exercise schedule for the most benefit. By alternating between resistance and aerobic exercise, you build muscle and burn fat.

DAY 1	DAY 2	DAY 3	DAY 4	DAY 5	DAY 6	DAY 7
Weight training in a fasted or fed state	Aerobic exercise or HIIT in a fasted state	Weight training in a fasted or fed state	Aerobic exercise or HIIT in a fasted state	Weight training in a fasted or fed state	Aerobic exercise or HIIT in a fasted state	Rest

Fasting Schedules for Young Women

When a woman is in the midst of her reproductive years (20s to 40s), she may have a goal of getting a lean body with a low body fat percentage (maybe even low enough to see her abs!). However, her body doesn't necessarily share that goal. As far as her body is concerned, now is the time to ensure that nutritional needs are being met. To make sure that happens, her body orchestrates hormonal changes that spur hunger and cravings at different times of the month, ensuring that nutrients will come in. What's a woman to do? Although the monthly hormonal shifts present challenges, this is a time for cooperation, not war. With an emphasis on proper nutrition and time-restricted eating, a woman can give her body what it needs and get what she wants.

The need to work with her body can be a frustrating thought. In a way, it seems like an extended fast, although challenging, would simplify life and get results. However, fasting for more than a day can disrupt the menstrual cycle, leading to unintentional outcomes in regards to reproductive health. The best approach is to practice shorter-term fasts interspersed with nutrient-rich eating windows. Examples of short-term fasts include 12 to 16 hours of fasting a day or modified alternate-day fasts.

Dr. Beckyism

Give your body what it needs, and it will give you what you want.

Be flexible with yourself. Follow different fasting routines throughout the month based on how you are feeling. If your hunger is elevated, a 12-hour fast will suffice for a day or two. If your hunger is low, fasting for 16 hours on consecutive days may be easy to do, enjoyable, and effective. At the end of the day, the important thing is to listen to your body and find the method that produces the results you want without negative consequences, such as disruption of your menstrual cycle, intensified hunger, mood swings, headaches, loss of mental clarity, or reduced energy.

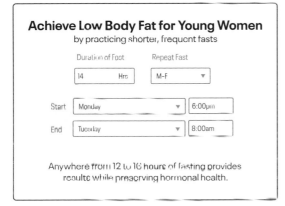

Achieve Low Body Fat for Young Women
by practicing shorter, frequent fasts

Duration of Fast	Repeat Fast
14 Hrs	M-F

Start | Monday | 6:00pm
End | Tuesday | 8:00am

Anywhere from 12 to 16 hours of fasting provides results while preserving hormonal health.

Nutritional considerations: Whichever fasting method you settle on, it is important to eat well during your eating window and avoid going too low in calories. Reducing your intake of sugar and refined grains gives you the most bang for your buck. But staying away from these tempting treats can be challenging with the hormonal swings that occur throughout the month. You can lessen cravings by eating in a way that stabilizes your blood sugar. As you'll learn in the next chapter, different foods affect your blood sugar level differently. By adding healthy fats to your diet and reducing refined carbs, you

stabilize your blood sugar and bypass the sugar crashes that lead to insatiable hunger that must be satisfied immediately. Consider adding a salad to your daily routine. The low-calorie, nutrient-dense vegetables in a salad provide volume and slow digestion. You can top your salad with high-quality fatty foods like salmon, hard-boiled eggs, cheese, avocados, nuts, and seeds. The fats add to the enjoyment of the meal and further stabilize your blood sugar to keep hunger and cravings under control.

Fasting Schedules for Stubborn Metabolisms

Some metabolisms require a bit more coaxing than others before they'll release fat. Genetics, existing health conditions, and advanced age are just a few of the things that can make it hard to lose weight. Fasting can tip the scale in your favor, but it will require a methodical approach with a few curveballs thrown in. Your body is a very adaptive machine. It will adjust to whatever you present it with, whether that change is good or bad. For instance, if you lift weights, your body will build muscle to withstand the stress. If you eat a low-calorie diet for too long, your body will adapt by lowering the number of calories you need. It can even adjust to a junk food diet, which explains why you feel worse before you feel better when you give up sugar. If you are someone who is slow to lose weight, your body may have found a steady state at which it is comfortable. Fasting can shake up your body's normal routine, forcing it to function differently, which can be just what you need to lose weight.

Fasting enhances your metabolism by increasing the production of metabolic regulators like norepinephrine and GH and boosting your level of NAD+, which is a vital substance needed for energy generation within your cells.[3] Fasting also makes you more metabolically flexible, which helps your body shift from running on sugar to running on fat. This flexibility comes about because fasting robs your body of its easy energy source (sugar), forcing it to create the enzymes and pathways needed to burn fat efficiently. In other words, fasting is a stress on your body, but it is a positive stress that creates a desired outcome. If you lose weight slowly or your weight has plateaued, it may help to throw your body a curveball by performing longer periods of fasting throughout the week. For instance, work your way up to the point that you can comfortably perform a 16-hour fast each day of the week and then choose a day to reduce your eating window to 4 hours, or try eating one meal a day. Although there is little research to support why this works, there are countless anecdotal stories from people who got the scale moving by periodically widening their fasting window.

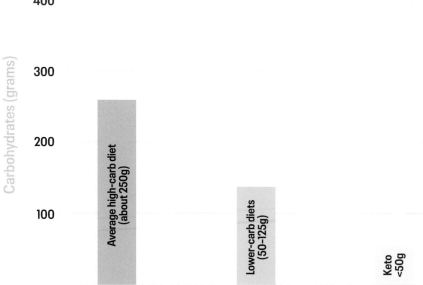

Ramp Up Your Metabolism
by varying your fasting schedule throughout the week

Duration of Fast	Repeat Fast
20 Hrs	M, W, F ▼

Start	Monday ▼	6:00pm
End	Tuesday ▼	2:00pm

To give your body an additional health advantage, eat a low-carb or keto diet.

Carbohydrate intake

Like fasting, a low-carb or very low-carb (keto) diet promotes fat loss by keeping your insulin level low.
If you have a stubborn metabolism, you may find that pairing IF with a low-carb or keto diet helps you lose weight.

Nutritional considerations: You can give your stubborn metabolism an additional kick in the pants by reducing your overall carb intake throughout the day. Carbohydrates are responsible for spiking the fat-storing hormone insulin. The average person eats around 250 grams or more of carbs a day with meals and snacks occurring every few hours. Those continual eating occasions keep insulin levels elevated and your metabolism locked in fat-storage mode. Like fasting, a low-carb diet disrupts this cycle by allowing time for your insulin level to drop. When it does, fatty acids stored in your fat cells can be released and burned for energy. Every person's metabolism is different, but most will find that cutting their carb intake in half makes it easier for them to lose weight. It also helps to focus on eating carbohydrates in their natural form, rather than refined. In other words, you want to consume carbs that resemble the living plant they came from. So eat vegetables, not veggie chips, and eat fruit, not fruit-flavored gummy snacks. You'll learn how to make healthy low-carb food choices in Chapter 6.

Fasting Schedules for Hectic Family and Work Calendars

Let's face it—life can be hectic at times. This frenzied pace can be a regular occurrence if you have kids at home, a demanding work schedule, or any other full calendar of commitments. If this is you, flexibility will be your main requirement when it comes to choosing a fasting method. Fortunately, you can still benefit from fasting, even if you

practice different methods throughout the week or simply skip meals when it's convenient. For instance, you may find that skipping breakfast is easy to do Monday through Friday as you shuffle kids out the door and rush to prepare for your workday, making a 16:8 fasting routine easy to do during the week, whereas the lack of structure on your weekends makes it feel more comfortable to eat normally. Your job can present you with scheduling challenges, from breakfast meetings to work that drags into the evening. If your work hours vary, vary your fasting times. Although there is evidence that eating earlier in the day and starting your fast at least 3 hours before bed is ideal, you will still gain benefits from a shortened eating window, no matter when that is.

This holds true for shift workers as well. Although working when the body is more inclined to sleep or shifting between day and evening work has notable disadvantages and health consequences, according to fasting researcher Dr. Satchin Panda, reducing your eating window has benefits. When rodents were kept awake and fed at a time that they would typically be sleeping, they still achieved benefits from time-restricted eating. In Dr. Panda's opinion, this finding could translate to human shift workers as long as they are able to get an adequate amount of sleep.[4] In other words, eating within a shortened eating window is superior to grazing all day long, even when your eating window occurs at a less-than-ideal time.

Fast fact: soda and your liver

Fatty liver, or more correctly nonalcoholic fatty liver disease (NAFLD), is just what you'd imagine from its name. It is the accumulation of fat in your liver that isn't caused by drinking alcohol. Considered the most common liver disease in Western societies, it's strongly influenced by a poor diet, in particular the consumption of soda.

A fatty liver develops when your liver takes nutrients from your diet and makes fat through a process called de novo lipogenesis. Through this process, your liver is making fat from things other than the fat you eat. That's the surprising part, right? Logic tells us that eating too much fat would cause the liver to store excess fat. Instead, what we see is that lipogenesis is driven by sugar and, more importantly, fructose in your diet. One of the main sources of fructose in the standard American diet is high-fructose corn syrup, which is found in regular soda. So kids and adults who drink a lot of soda have a high risk for developing fatty liver.

A fatty liver is an inefficient liver. Your liver is your detox organ and essential for an efficiently running metabolism. In its early stages, the progression of fatty liver can be halted with corrections to your diet and lifestyle. If not caught early, fatty liver can progress to nonalcoholic steatohepatitis (NASH), which can lead to scarring or cirrhosis of the liver. The takeaway: if you cut soda and drinks sweetened with high fructose corn syrup or sugar out of your diet, then you'll have a happier liver that is more than willing to help you move toward your goal.

Stay on Top of Your Schedule
by fasting when it works for you

Duration of Fast		Repeat Fast	
16	Hrs	Any day ▼	

Start	Monday ▼	6:30pm
End	Tuesday ▼	10:30am

Skip meals when you're too busy to eat.

Nutritional considerations: Because life is busy, you'll want to look at the big picture when it comes to nutrition and tackle the biggest problems first. This includes cutting out sugary drinks, swapping healthy snacks for unhealthy ones, and finding nutritious meals that can make it to the table quickly.

The action that will give you the most robust health and weight-loss return is cutting out soda and energy drinks. With nothing to slow its absorption, these sugary drinks cause a quick spike in blood sugar and insulin, promoting weight gain, inflammation, and disease. Diet soda and sugar-free energy drinks are not healthy alternatives and should also be avoided. However, if they help you break your sugar habit, they can be used as a temporary stepping stone to ending your addiction.

You can improve grab-and-go snacks dramatically with very little effort. For example, fill a baggie with raw almonds and keep it in your purse or car. They last for a long time, and the mix of healthy fat and protein make them an ideal swap for a vending machine bag of chips. Candy bars and baked goods will call to you if you let yourself get too hungry, so stock your work and home fridge with healthier alternatives like chopped veggies, pre-sliced cheese, and hard-boiled eggs.

Another challenge for busy individuals is finding quick and easy meals for dinner. Although it can be tempting to pull into the drive-thru, order a pizza, or tear open a box of mac 'n' cheese, filling your body with these low-nutritional-value foods can negate the benefits you achieve through fasting. There are many ways to get quick meals on the table. For instance, many grocery stores have fully stocked salad bars, ready-to-eat rotisserie chicken, and other pre-cooked meats (just avoid breaded items). Eggs can be scrambled or fried for a quick and tasty dinner, and if you must pick up a fast-food meal, choose a ready-made salad. Your body will thank you for the nutritional boost, and you will be rewarded with another step toward your goal.

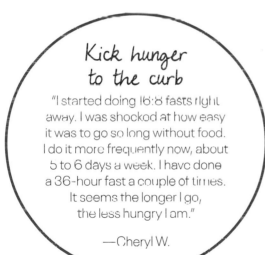

Kick hunger to the curb

"I started doing 16:8 fasts right away. I was shocked at how easy it was to go so long without food. I do it more frequently now, about 5 to 6 days a week. I have done a 36-hour fast a couple of times. It seems the longer I go, the less hungry I am."

—Cheryl W.

Fasting Schedules for Renewed Health

Are you looking at fasting as a way to rejuvenate your health? As we learned, fasting has many benefits beyond weight loss, from fixing blood sugar disorders, to improving your cholesterol profile, to boosting mental clarity. Fasting can enhance the quality of your life in other ways as well. According to the study, by adhering to a daily 16-hour fast for 4 weeks, 10 overweight men and women over the age of 65 with limited mobility lost an average of 5.7 pounds (2.6kg), and improved their walking speed by a clinically significant amount.[5]

As we age, biological changes contribute to a progressive decline in mental and physical function that can eventually rob us of our independence. A poor diet, excess weight, and a sedentary lifestyle accelerate these changes. Low-calorie diets have proven to be effective for increasing longevity, reducing cardiac risk factors, and improving insulin sensitivity. Despite these health benefits, most people have difficulty sticking with calorie restriction over the long term.

Fasting offers an alternative. Fasting leads to similar benefits, and many people find it easier to stick with than traditional low-calorie diets. To achieve the results you're after, timing and consistency will be the factors you need to get the results you want. A study mentioned in Chapter 3 showed that men with prediabetes who ate early and started their fast at 3pm were able to improve insulin sensitivity, lower their blood pressure, and reduce oxidative stress, even without weight loss.[6]

Dr. Beckyism

If you have an unplanned splurge, get right back on track with your next meal, not the next day.

Most of the studies looking at fasting for improved health required participants to stick to their fasting routines for weeks or months at a time. Because it takes time for the body to heal itself, you'll be happiest with your results if you look at fasting as a long-term strategy. With your doctor's okay, practice a time-restricted eating schedule and stick with that routine for a few months. If you take medication that must be taken with food or if you feel better with breakfast, it may be easier for you to fast for 14 hours of the day. If not, work up to the point that you feel comfortable fasting for 16 hours a day. Also, you may be able to get an additional health boost by eating early rather than late. Consider ending your eating day by 5pm or earlier. If you're looking to improve blood work results, have your blood tested before starting your fasting routine and then retest it in a few months to evaluate your progress.

Rejuvenate Your Health
by getting an early start to your fast

Duration of Fast	Repeat Fast
16 Hrs	Daily ▼

Start	Monday ▼	5:00pm
End	Tuesday ▼	9:00am

To give your body an additional health advantage, end your eating window by 5pm.

Nutritional considerations: Although fasting can counter many of the biological changes that promote mental and physical decline, it can't correct all of them. That's why, when it comes to rejuvenating your health, what you eat is as important as when you eat.

Your body needs nutrients to repair damage, but if your current diet is high in nutrient-poor foods (e.g., packaged convenience foods, sugar, and fried foods), changing your diet can feel like a daunting task. To make the transition go smoothly, it helps to *add* before you *subtract*. By strategically adding high-quality foods before you remove the junk, you quiet sugar withdrawal symptoms, limit cravings, and maintain your mental clarity and energy level.

A good first step is to add low-calorie, nutrient-dense vegetables to your daily diet. Aim to have a large salad for lunch, and add a large portion of cooked vegetables to your plate at dinner. With those additions in place, you can subtract the biggest health menace, which is sugar. Avoid stirring sugar into drinks or sprinkling it on food, and check labels. If a food has sugar listed as one of the top three ingredients, leave it on the shelf. Getting the veggies in and the sugar out will go a long way toward improving your health. You can propel your health even further by adding whole foods as you eliminate processed and refined foods. A practical way to do this is to start eating more meals at home. Many grab-and-go meals and fast foods are cooked in unhealthy oils and filled with refined ingredients that digest quickly. Cooking meals at home puts you in control of your diet and your health.

OPTIMIZING YOUR HEALTH: FASTING + DIET

There is no better goal to pursue than good health. It is what allows you to be prepared for life's unexpected moments and age with grace. Fasting is a versatile tool that can be used to improve your body composition, spark weight loss, and rejuvenate your health. It will get you far on your journey, but why not maximize your results by adding a healthy diet to your fasting strategy? As it turns out, improving your diet is as easy as 0-1-2-3.... Turn to the next chapter to discover my diet food strategy that makes healthy eating easy and unintimidating.

6

WHAT SHOULD YOU EAT?

What lies ahead

- **Make 0-1-2-3 your daily foundation for healthy living.** This means 0 grams of added sugar; 1 large salad; 2 cups of cooked nonstarchy vegetables; and 3 hours before bed, stop eating.

- **A low-carb, high-fat diet is an effective way to stabilize your blood sugar and control hunger.** This combination makes it easier to fast.

- **Learn how to break your fast.** For fasting patterns that last less than a day, you can break your fast with a normal meal. For longer fasts, you'll avoid digestive issues by reintroducing food slowly.

You've chosen your fasting routine. Now it's time to maximize your results with a healthy diet. What to eat for better health is a complex web, but there are some universal rules that simplify healthy eating. My 0–1–2–3 strategy shares four of those rules. I like to say that by following the four daily habits that make up this strategy, you give your body no choice but to lose weight. In this chapter, you'll learn why I say that and how to build on the foundational rules to accelerate your results.

0-1-2-3: YOUR FOUNDATION FOR HEALTHY EATING

Figuring out how to eat for better health and weight control can feel like a daunting task, but the road to healthy eating starts with four simple rules. These straightforward guidelines can be folded into any diet strategy, from a high-quality vegan diet to a well-formulated keto diet, so you don't need to change your diet preferences to employ them. When you follow these rules on a daily basis, they stabilize your blood sugar, which steadies insulin, encourages weight loss, and controls hunger, so fasting is easier. I use a simple acronym—0–1–2–3—to help you remember the rules. Here is what it stands for:

0 grams of added sugar
1 large salad
2 cups of cooked nonstarchy vegetables
3 hours before bed, stop eating

Reaching your health or weight-loss goal may require more than these four changes. We will do a deeper dive into healthy eating as we progress through this chapter, but these rules serve as a foundation for healthy eating. If you ever stray from your diet, 0–1–2–3 will get you back on track quickly. Let's learn more about each element of the strategy and how you can get them working for you.

How 0-1-2-3 enhances your fasting experience

* When you remove sugar from your diet, you stabilize your blood sugar and insulin levels, which promotes fat loss and controls hunger.

* Eating multiple servings of nonstarchy vegetables physically and biochemically fills you up, which further controls hunger.

* Declaring an end to your eating window 3 hours before bed kick-starts your fast, eliminates mindless snacking, and improves the quality of your sleep.

Breaking Free from Sugar

The first rule of the 0–1–2–3 strategy instructs you to stop eating sugar (0g added sugar), which admittedly is a scary proposition because sugar is everywhere and it's highly addictive. The average person consumes about 17 teaspoons of sugar a day, from the obvious addition of table sugar in things like coffee, tea, and cereal, to the ingestion of hidden sugars in "healthy foods" like salad dressings, yogurt, and fruit drinks.

That translates into a yearly total of about 57 pounds (26kg) of sugar per person.[1] All of that sugar is wreaking havoc with our health, yet it keeps calling to us because it is an addictive substance. When you eat sugar, a feel-good chemical called *dopamine* is released into a part of your brain called the *nucleus accumbens*. This area of your brain is nicknamed the pleasure or reward center because when it's stimulated, you feel good. (This is the same part of your brain, by the way, that is stimulated by cocaine.) In other words, when you eat sugar, your brain says, "Wow! That was great! Give me some more of that." So you can see what you're up against when you try to give up sugar, and here I am telling you to give it up!

I am the first to admit that it is not easy to break free from the powerful grip of sugar. In my younger years, I was thoroughly addicted to sugar, and I have the cavities to prove it. In those days, the thought of living without sugar seemed unrealistic. I would wake up with sugar on my mind and go to bed with the same thoughts racing through my head. It ruled my life and took over my focus. Today, I lead a mostly sugar-free life with rare exceptions like pumpkin pie at Thanksgiving (non-negotiable) and the occasional piece of birthday cake. Despite those few indulgences, sugar rarely tempts me anymore, and I pass it by with little effort. I can attest, as can many of the people I have coached to a sugar-free life, that there is freedom, energy, and mental clarity on the other side of sugar. My motto today is that if I am going to eat something, it not only has to taste good, but it must also leave me feeling good after I eat it. If not, then it's not worth it. Sugar sure tastes good, but that moment of pleasure sends my blood sugar on a roller-coaster ride that eventually zaps my energy and leaves me ravenously hungry for another sugar fix. Eating sugar is not worth the price you pay, so how do you break free, and what does leading a sugar-free life look like?

Dr. Beckyism

For me, chocolate does nothing but make me want more chocolate.

How to get sugar out of your life: You'll want to stop adding table sugar to foods and drinks and avoid items with sugar (or one of its many aliases) listed as one of the top three ingredients (see *Alternate-names for sugar* on page 87). The cruel joke is that breaking free from sugar comes with a price tag. Like other addictive substances, when you give up sugar, your body goes through withdrawal, leaving you with a few days of irritability, fatigue, headaches, and cravings.

Sugar has no redeeming qualities and can overtake your life, but only if you let it. Here are some things that I've found helpful for quitting sugar:

- **Understand that sugar addiction is real.** There is no shame in wanting to eat sugar, and you're not weak or pathetic for being drawn to it.
- **Set up a short-term goal.** Telling yourself that you can never eat sugar again is an overwhelming thought that can backfire. Instead, set a goal to give up sugar for 1 day, and then step it up to 1 week, and so on.

- **Fill up on foods that stabilize your blood sugar.** It is the dips in blood sugar that bring on that intense hunger that's hard to dismiss. By filling up on nonstarchy vegetables, healthy fats, and protein, you prevent the dips and stay in control.

- **Cut out soda and sugary drinks.** With almost 11 teaspoons of sugar in a 12-ounce can, soda is responsible for much of the sugar consumption in the average diet.[1] Juice can be equally as bad. Even if there is no sugar added, juice contains all of the sugar from the fruit without the fiber to slow its absorption.

- **Sugar substitutes like Equal, monk fruit, Splenda, stevia, and xylitol can be used as a temporary crutch to help ease yourself away from sugar.** However, they will keep your sweet tooth alive and kicking. You'll be happiest with your health and hunger control if you wean yourself off of them as you progress on your diet.

- **Avoid extreme hunger.** If you let yourself get too hungry as you transition to a sugar-free life, your body will try to get you to eat by spiking cravings. If you struggle with giving up sugar, start with a 12-hour fast until you feel more in control.

- **Cut your sweet tooth with mint.** Do you ever have a feeling that you want "a little something sweet" after a meal? If so, change the taste in your mouth by brushing your teeth with a minty toothpaste or popping a stick of sugar-free gum in your mouth. I call these tricks "stoppers," and you can learn more in the *Fast fact* below.

Fast fact: using stoppers

The mere act of eating can stimulate your appetite, making it hard to stop. To close your eating window without overeating, try using a "stopper." A stopper is an item, drink, or activity that allows you to separate from eating. Here are three stoppers I use:

* **Chewing gum.** Place a stick of minty sugar-free gum in your mouth as soon as you are done with a meal. The bold flavor will change the taste in your mouth, making it unappealing to continue eating.

* **Floss.** Keep a package of dental floss in your TV room. If you feel like snacking during your favorite program, floss instead. Your mouth will feel fresh and clean, removing any inclination to dirty it up with more food. Brushing your teeth also works!

* **Hot beverages.** Drink hot coffee or tea because it takes time to drink, which gives your brain time to realize that you're full. Pour a cup after a meal or in the afternoon, and you'll naturally move away from a desire to eat.

Alternate names for sugar

Sometimes sugar is easy to spot, and sometimes it's not.

Sugar can go by many alternative names. If any of the following sugar aliases are listed as one of the first three ingredients, leave the item on the shelf.

Nutrition Facts	%DV* amount per 1 cup		%DV* amount per 1 cup		*The % Daily Values (DV) tells you how much a nutrient in a serving of food contributes to a daily diet. 2000 calories a day is used for general nutrition advice.
9 servings Serving Size 1 cup (33g)	9%	**Total Fat** 1.5g	9%	**Total Carbs** 27g	
	5%	Saturated Fat 1g	0%	Dietary Fiber 2g	
		Trans Fat 0g		Sugars 13g	
120 Calories per cup	0%	**Cholesterol** 0g		Added 10g	
	12%	**Sodium** 280mg		**Protein** 0g	

0% Vitamin D 0mcg • 6% Calcium 80mg • 6% Iron 1mg • 10% Potassium 470mg • 15% Thiamin 0.2mg • 8% Riboflavin 0.1mg • 10% Niacin 1.6mg

INGREDIENTS: enriched flour (wheat flour, niacin, reduced iron, thiamin mononitrate, riboflavin, folic acid), corn syrup, (sugar,) soybean and palm oil, corn syrup solids, dextrose, high fructose corn syrup, fructose, glycerin, contains 2% or less of cocoa, modified corn starch, salt, calcium carbonate

Common alternative names for sugar:

* Cane sugar
* Corn syrup
* Dextrose
* Fructose
* Fruit juice concentrate
* High-fructose corn syrup
* Maltodextrin

Less common (but equally sneaky) names for sugar:

* Agave nectar
* Barley malt
* Evaporated cane juice
* Glucose
* Maltose
* Molasses
* Sucrose

Adding a Salad to Your Daily Diet

The second rule of the 0–1–2–3 strategy asks you to eat one large salad every day. Does that sound boring? I get how a bowl of lettuce with a few veggies and some store-bought dressing can be unappealing, but that would be an inaccurate illustration of this rule. There is an art to assembling a delicious salad, and you can master it even if you hate to cook. When you have this skill down pat, you fill your body with high-volume nutrient-rich foods that stabilize your blood sugar, helping you sail through your fasting hours with ease. It's time to get a fresh perspective on salads as hearty meals.

How to build a better salad: Your daily salad should be thought of as a meal. You can break your fast with a salad at lunch or, if you prefer, eat it at dinnertime. The base of your salad can be 2 to 4 cups of leafy greens (about 100–150g), with darker leafy greens being the most nutritious. Top your salad with assorted nonstarchy vegetables like tomatoes, onions, and peppers, and make it a hearty meal with the addition of healthy fats and protein. The healthy fats you get from protein-rich foods like raw nuts and seeds, hard-boiled eggs, chicken, steak, cheese, and avocados further stabilize your blood sugar and help you to absorb the fat-soluble vitamins from the vegetables. Salad dressing can also add to the taste and health value of your salad, but there are a lot of ways to go wrong with salad dressing. If you use a store-bought brand, be sure to read the ingredients list. Look out for added sugar or high-fructose corn syrup, as well as unhealthy vegetable oils such as soybean oil, which is high in inflammation-promoting omega-6 fatty acids. To avoid harmful ingredients, you can make your own salad dressing—you'll find some great recipes in Part 2!

Dr. Becky's typical salad

Here is the lunchtime salad that I have on a typical day. This high-fat salad satisfies my hunger for hours. If I'm in the mood for a bit of natural sweetness, I add a few slices of an apple.

Serves: 1

Ingredients

2–4 cups (128g) mixed salad greens (such as spring mix)

½ avocado (68g), sliced

3 tbsp (28g) feta cheese crumbles

2 tbsp (13g) chopped raw walnuts

2 tbsp (18g) raw sunflower seeds

1½ tbsp (23ml) full-fat salad dressing (such as Primal Kitchen brand, or homemade with oil and vinegar)

Instructions

Combine all ingredients in a bowl, and enjoy!

NUTRITION PER SERVING

Calories **504** · Fat **45** · Carbohydrates **18g** · Fiber **9g** · Protein **13g**

A Daily Side of Veggies

The "2" of the 0–1–2–3 strategy stands for 2 cups of cooked nonstarchy vegetables, which is a portion size equal to two fists. To fulfill this rule, you'll be eating a large portion of veggies mixed into recipes or as a side dish with one of your daily meals. Nonstarchy vegetables refer to foods like broccoli, cauliflower, asparagus, snap peas, green beans, onions, mushrooms, and zucchini—not corn and potatoes, which are starchy vegetables. If you are someone who has a hard time losing weight, you'll find that you do best if you stick with the nonstarchy choices. I recommend cooked vegetables for variety, but the main value of a daily salad and side of vegetables is that you fill up your body both physically and biochemically, making your fasting experience much more enjoyable. The physical volume from the veggies takes a long time to digest, keeping hunger at bay for hours. The flood of vitamins and minerals tells your body and brain that your nutrient needs have been met, so there is no need for more.

You'll find that the vegetable-heavy meals and side dishes in Part 2 will keep things interesting. However, if cooking is not your thing, simplify life by opening a bag of frozen vegetables and cooking them in boiling water. When they're cooked, don't shy away from adding fat. Butter, olive oil, nuts, and seeds enhance the flavor of the vegetables and help your body absorb the nutrients.

The 3-Hour Rule

The last rule of the strategy instructs you to stop eating 3 hours before bed. Not eating in the evening hours does many things:

- It allows the level of glucose and insulin in your blood to remain low overnight, which promotes fat burning.

- It eliminates mindless late-night snacking, which can save you hundreds of calories.

- It improves your sleep because your body is not shuttling blood flow to your digestive tract, which elevates your core temperature and interferes with sleep.

To enhance your results, I recommend that you set a regular time each night to stop eating. To do this, simply take a moment to think about what the clock says right before you shut off your nightstand lamp and close your eyes. Do you have a time in mind? Great! Now, subtract 3 hours and note that time as the end of your eating window and the beginning of your fast.

0-1-2-3 works!

"I have spent the last 6 years trying to get rid of menopausal weight gain and a thick middle. I have been following Dr. Becky's 0-1-2-3 strategy for weight loss for 80 days now, and I have lost 15lbs and inches off my waist! I watched her videos, followed her recipes (minus the red meat and chicken, just fish), minimal workouts (just walking and small movements with weights), and no eating 3 hours before bedtime. I am so happy with my results. I am back down to 129lbs. (I am turning 60 years old very soon and I haven't been at this weight for over 12 years!)"

—S. Fredrick

THE REST OF YOUR EATING STRATEGY: A MACRO PROFILE LOW IN CARBS

Abiding by the 0-1-2-3 rules will get you far along the path to better health and weight loss, but there are other foods in the world than sugar and vegetables. To fill in the blanks and put together a complete eating strategy, let's go back to what we know. Earlier in the book, we learned that there are three macronutrients that provide us with calories: carbohydrates, fats, and proteins. If health were simple, you could ingest those nutrients in equal portions and call it a day. Unfortunately, this simplistic model, which we've followed for decades, has a couple of glaring flaws. It assumes that all calories are equal and food quality doesn't matter. With this assumption, 100 calories of cake equals 100 calories of meat, which equals 100 calories of salad. The assumption continued with the thought being that all of these calories are dumped into a collective bucket at the same rate, and there they sit until you need a bit of energy. As long as you didn't overeat, you'd control your weight and be healthy. This model seemed logical, but it didn't seem to work, as evidenced by the soaring obesity rates of the past decades. The reason it doesn't work is because calories are not simply dumped into a collective bucket inside your body. Instead, the calories that are not used immediately are directed into separate storage containers and stored as either readily available glycogen or hard-to-access fat. The filling of those storage containers is controlled by a hormone with which you are now familiar—insulin.

Yep! Insulin was the game-changer in our understanding of how fat is gained and lost. If you eat in a way that spikes insulin, your body quickly fills the small glycogen stores and then converts the remaining energy to fat. If you eat in a way that keeps insulin low, you create an internal environment that promotes fat release. Eating no food (fasting) is one way to keep insulin low; making smart food choices is another.

What we now know is that the calories we get from carbs, fat, and protein are not alike. They have vastly different effects on blood sugar and insulin levels. Carbohydrates cause the most significant spike in insulin, protein provides a moderate rise, and fat produces little or no increase in insulin. With this understanding, it makes sense to eat a low-carb, high-fat, moderate-protein diet. For some of you, this way of eating sounds completely counter to what you've learned in the past. I agree that it takes the familiar food pyramid and turns it upside down. However, if weight loss has been hard for you,

Calories are not created equal

When you eat, insulin is produced in different amounts depending on the macronutrient breakdown of your food. Carbs cause the greatest spike in insulin, while fat has little or no impact.[2]

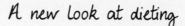

A new look at dieting

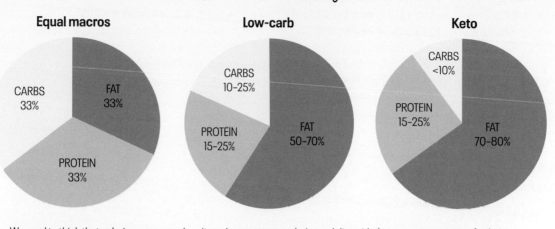

Equal macros

CARBS 33%
FAT 33%
PROTEIN 33%

Low-carb

CARBS 10–25%
PROTEIN 15–25%
FAT 50–70%

Keto

CARBS <10%
PROTEIN 15–25%
FAT 70–80%

We used to think that calories were equal, so it made sense to eat a balanced diet with the same percentage of calories coming from fat, protein, and carbohydrates. We now know that each macronutrient affects blood sugar and insulin levels differently. Because carbs cause the highest spike in blood sugar/insulin and fat has the least impact, a low-carb, high-fat diet helps you lose weight.

I think you will find that controlling your blood sugar and insulin level by eating in this way tips the scale in your favor and keeps your hunger under control. Eating for stable blood sugar and hunger control is the basis of low-carb and keto diets.

If there is one culprit that we can point our finger at in the upward trend of obesity, it's the overloading of refined carbohydrates in our diet. Yet these quick-absorbing foods have been flying under the radar for years because we were so focused on the falsely accused dietary fats. If you're like me, you grew up with the mindset that eating fat made you fat, and if you wanted to control your weight, you should swap out the fats for carbs. This idea of cutting fat and boosting carbs made sense for many reasons. First, carbohydrates are a quick and easy source of energy for your body. Also, gram for gram, fat has more than two times the

calories of carbs. So the weight-loss formula that made sense on paper was that weight loss should happen when you replace fat with carbs, employ a bit of willpower to control portions, and burn off excess energy through exercise. A good thought, but problematic.

Food energy sources

Energy source	Calories per gram
Fats	9
Proteins	4
Carbohydrates	4

Gram for gram, fat has more than two times the calories of carbs. However, carbs cause more of a spike in blood sugar and insulin than fat.

Problem number 1 that dooms the low-fat, high-carb promise is the lack of evident effectiveness: we all get fatter eating this way, as evidenced by the familiar obesity maps that show how obesity has skyrocketed over the past decades. Problem number 2 is that many people cannot follow this simple formula for very long because it makes you hungry. Carbs are quick energy, but they burn up quickly, much like twigs on a fire. You get a short burst of energy, but if you want to keep your fire burning, you must continually eat to stoke the fire. If you don't, your body reminds you to do so by making you crave carbs, and the cycle repeats itself, leaving you with the need to eat every couple of hours. After years of trying to "do the right thing," we fell into this collective mindset that those who could not lose weight either lacked willpower or lied about what they were eating. In reality, the flaw is in the equation.

Despite its flaws, there are those who do well and enjoy a low-fat diet. For a disciplined person, a low-fat diet that is filled with high-quality, unprocessed carbs works. However, because carbohydrates encompass such a wide range of foods, adhering to this style of eating requires quite a bit of police work. To replace the flavor that is lost,

Prevalence of obesity in the U.S. population

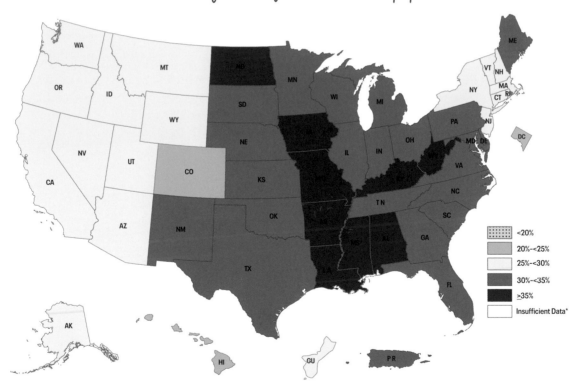

▦	<20%
▨	20%–<25%
▢	25%–<30%
▓	30%–<35%
■	≥35%
□	Insufficient Data*

In the United States from 1999–2000 through 2017–2018, the prevalence of obesity increased from 30.5 percent to 42.4 percent, and the prevalence of severe obesity increased from 4.7 percent to 9.2 percent.[3, 4]

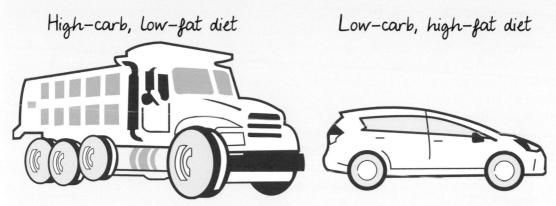

High-carb, low-fat diet

Low-carb, high-fat diet

Eating a high-carb diet is much like driving a big truck that is not fuel-efficient. The vehicle has a lot of power and energy, but it needs to stop at the gas station often to refuel. When you cut carbs, your metabolism runs more like a fuel-efficient hybrid vehicle. When fuel is not coming in from your diet, your metabolism can shift to running on its alternative fuel, which is fat. You experience sustained energy all day long with less need to refuel or eat.

foods that are made to be lower in fat often add sugar or a sugar alternative that can spike insulin and block fat loss, making it imperative that you read labels in search of unhealthy ingredients.

Lowering your carbohydrate intake, and in particular your refined carb intake, can be done regardless of whether you prefer an animal- or plant-based diet. Lower-carb diets are slowly but surely gaining acceptance because they work not only for weight loss but also for better health. A study involving a group of individuals with type 2 diabetes found that following a low-carb diet for 1 year allowed the average study participant to lower their HbA1c from 7.6 to 6.3 percent, lose 12 percent of their body weight, and reduce their use of diabetes medication.[5]

In a nutshell, to control blood sugar and insulin, improve your health, and lose weight, do the following:

- Limit your carbohydrate intake.

- Get the majority of your calories from healthy fats.

- Consume an adequate but moderate amount of protein.

Let's look at what each of these elements looks like in real life.

The Hierarchy of Carbs

Carbs are not created equal. Some cause weight gain while others flood your body with the nutrients it needs to keep your metabolism running strong. It goes without saying that sugar tops the list of unhealthy carbs, but what if the sugar is mixed with other things like flour, oil, or maybe an egg to make bread, pasta, cereal, or crackers? Some of those foods have visible evidence of healthy ingredients. For example, pasta made with spinach has a green color, and whole-wheat bread often has visible grains and seeds baked in. Are they better choices? You can argue that because there are remnants of whole grains and natural ingredients present that it takes longer for your body to break down the food. If weight loss is your goal, however, these processed foods (and more obvious junk foods like cookies, cakes, and candies) hold little value because they are still highly refined. It is the refining process that makes the food lose value. When a whole food goes through the refining process, the parts of the original plant that are prone to spoilage are removed. This increases the shelf life, which is why a box of pasta can sit in your pantry for years, yet cook up as if you just bought it yesterday. Unfortunately, the parts of the plant that are prone to rot are also the parts that contain fiber, nutrients, and often the flavor.

When evaluating carbs for their health value, we can take a step up from refined carbs and look at fruit and starchy plant foods, such as quinoa, rice, beans, oats, corn, and potatoes. These foods contain vitamins and minerals that benefit your body. If your metabolism is strong and you are young and active, these whole carbs have a place in your diet. However, if you are someone who has trouble losing weight, you may find that the natural sugar and starch in these foods make it hard for your body to lose weight. If you are slow to lose weight or have a long history of eating a poor diet or being overweight, you'll be happiest with your weight loss if you reduce your fruit and starch intake and focus on nonstarchy vegetables as your carb source.

Following a Low-Carb Diet

As you can see, a wide range of foods contain carbs. To follow a low-carb diet, you will need to track how many carbs you're eating in a day. If you are someone with a relatively robust metabolism who can handle fruits and starchy carbs, then a low-carb meal plan should work for you. If you are someone with a broken metabolism or a lot of weight to lose, then a keto meal plan may work the best for you.

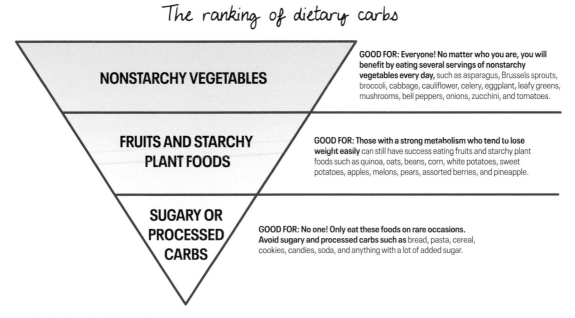

The ranking of dietary carbs

NONSTARCHY VEGETABLES

GOOD FOR: Everyone! No matter who you are, you will benefit by eating several servings of nonstarchy vegetables every day, such as asparagus, Brussels sprouts, broccoli, cabbage, cauliflower, celery, eggplant, leafy greens, mushrooms, bell peppers, onions, zucchini, and tomatoes.

FRUITS AND STARCHY PLANT FOODS

GOOD FOR: Those with a strong metabolism who tend to lose weight easily can still have success eating fruits and starchy plant foods such as quinoa, oats, beans, corn, white potatoes, sweet potatoes, apples, melons, pears, assorted berries, and pineapple.

SUGARY OR PROCESSED CARBS

GOOD FOR: No one! Only eat these foods on rare occasions. Avoid sugary and processed carbs such as bread, pasta, cereal, cookies, candies, soda, and anything with a lot of added sugar.

The continuum of carbs in your diet

PERCENTAGE OF CARBS IN YOUR DAILY CALORIC INTAKE

	10%		25%

KETO:
Less than 10% of daily calories as carbs (less than 50g per day).
Those with stubborn metabolisms who have difficulty with weight loss will find success eating within a keto range.

LOW-CARB:
10-25% of daily calories as carbs (50-125g per day).
Those with responsive metabolisms who lose weight relatively easily will recognize better health within this low-carb range.

MODERATE- TO HIGH-CARB:
More than 25% of daily calories as carbs (more than 125g per day).
A diet exceeding 25% of calories as carbs will require more police work to limit the quick-digesting carbs that spike insulin.

There is no official definition of a low-carb or keto diet, but the consensus is as follows: a low-carb diet is between 10 and 25 percent of your daily calorie intake as carbohydrates (about 50–125g per day), and a ketogenic diet is less than 10 percent of your daily calorie intake as carbohydrates (less than 50g per day).

Dr. Beckyism

You cannot outrun the metabolic impact of a poor diet.

You can see that a keto diet is simply a very low-carb diet. If you are just getting started, I recommend that you aim to take in 100 to 125 grams of carbs a day and monitor your results. If you feel good and you are consistently losing weight, then great! You've found a level that works for you. If you are not losing weight as desired, you may find that you need to drop your carb intake lower or into the keto range.

Fast fact: fat and refined carbs don't mix

Is there a lethal combination that makes a food irresistible?

A study published in 2015 had participants rank foods from most to least addictive. They found the following foods to be highly addictive:

* Pizza
* Chocolate
* Chips
* Cookies
* Ice cream
* French fries
* Cheeseburgers
* Regular soda
* Cake

It might not surprise you that these foods made the list, but what is it about them that makes them so hard to resist? Take a closer look, and you'll notice that they share three characteristics: (1) they are refined carbs, (2) they have a high glycemic load, which means that they spike your blood sugar, (3) and they contain fat. When combined, these factors make a food irresistible.[11]

Following a High-Fat Diet

When you cut carbs, you need to replace the lost calories with foods that will satisfy your body. Fats are very satisfying foods, and when you learn how to get the right types and amounts of fats into your diet, you keep hunger under control and unlock your body's fat-burning metabolism. However, adding fat presents a mental hurdle because of the pervasive belief that eating fat makes you fat. We need to be clear—the fat in our diets does not automatically become fat on our bodies. A study published in *The American Journal of Medicine,* which bears the hard-to-misinterpret title "Dietary Fat Is Not a Major Determinant of Body Fat," showed that fat consumption within the range of 18 to 40 percent of the body's energy needs had little if any effect on body fatness.[6] Surprisingly, sugar from carbohydrates causes the liver to make most of the fats floating around in your blood.[7] As it turns out, time has shown that the substantial decline in the percentage of energy obtained from dietary fat has corresponded with a sharp increase in the prevalence of obesity.[6] Moreover, there is evidence that a ketogenic diet, which is a very low-carb, high-fat diet, suppresses appetite, helping you stretch out the hours between meals.[8, 9]

The bottom line is that it's time to kick low-fat muffins, yogurts, and crackers to the curb; fats are back in style. Let me correct that—*healthy* fats are in style; bad fats belong in the garbage can. Like carbs, there are healthy and unhealthy choices when it comes to fats.

I recommend at least 50 percent of your calories come from healthy fats, which are natural fats from whole foods. Unhealthy fats are processed or man-made lab creations.

Healthy fats:

*   Avocados
*   Cooking fats (butter, lard, tallow)
*   Eggs
*   Fatty fish
*   Full-fat dairy
*   High-quality meats
*   Nuts and seeds
*   Oils (coconut oil, olive oil, avocado oil)

Unhealthy fats:

*   Fake fats (margarine, Crisco, shortening)
*   Trans fats (hydrogenated fats)
*   Vegetable oils (canola oil, corn oil, grapeseed oil, peanut oil, soybean oil, safflower oil, sunflower oil, cottonseed oil)

With their healthy-sounding name, it might surprise you that vegetable oils are unhealthy fats. Despite their virtuous name, many vegetable oils are high in inflammatory omega-6 fatty acids and extracted using harmful chemicals or heat that causes them to degrade. Decades ago, vegetable oils were heralded as heart-healthy fats, but today we know this advice is dead wrong. These refined oils create inflammation and oxidize or degrade cholesterol in your body, making heart disease more likely.[10]

Following a Moderate Protein Diet

Because of the many uses of protein in your body, it is essential that you bring it in through your diet. However, when it comes to protein, there is a balancing act—get too little and your body doesn't have the raw materials it needs to build and repair tissues, but get too much and you could be opening the door to potential health risks. How much your health is negatively affected by a high protein intake is a controversial topic. However, we do know that overconsumption of protein causes an insulin response that could impact your body's ability to burn fat.

Inside your digestive tract, protein is broken down into amino acids that get sent to your bloodstream. These basic building blocks can then be linked back together to make things like enzymes, hormones, and muscle fibers. As your body uses up the amino acids, you need to replenish the supply by eating protein-containing foods. But let's say that you take in 100 grams of protein and only need 75 of those grams for growth and repair. What happens to the excess protein? Some of the surplus will be excreted, but some gets converted to glucose in your liver through a process called *gluconeogenesis*. If this newly made glucose is not needed for immediate energy, it must go into storage, with much of it being escorted to your fat cells. In other words, excess protein isn't stored as protein; it's stored as fat.

A moderate intake of protein will meet the needs of most people. Protein requirements may be higher for older individuals and those who are physically active or recovering from a significant illness. If you experience fatigue or hunger that lasts more than a few days or you are a vegetarian who avoids animal sources of protein (e.g., eggs and fish), you may find that adding more protein-containing foods or a protein supplement is beneficial.

A moderate level of protein is reached when protein makes up about 15 to 25 percent of your daily caloric intake. If you are eating 1,400 calories a day, that works out to 210 to 350 calories (about 52–88g) of protein per day. Foods that contain a good amount of protein include eggs, meat, fish, poultry, and dairy products. Other sources include beans, nuts, seeds, unrefined whole grains, and certain vegetables.

DO CALORIES MATTER?

Many of the fasting studies performed on animals and people revealed a shocking finding: by merely reducing the number of hours during which participants consumed food, they lost weight and improved their health. On top of that, many of the fasting methods that you learned about in Chapter 4 put no restrictions on what or how much you can eat during your eating window. So are calories unimportant? Can you truly eat with abandon and reap the benefits? The answer to that question requires us to look a bit closer into the research. Participants in research studies are monitored to ensure that they are sticking with the fasting guidelines established by the research team. These studies are carried out over several weeks or months, which means that the participants are fasting daily for long periods. So one has to ask: is consistency a key component? As I mentioned before, the human body is very good at adapting to the routine it is presented. If you have been a regular breakfast eater in the past, your body adjusts to your routine and produces digestive enzymes and triggers hunger hormones in anticipation of the meal. If you switch up your routine by skipping breakfast, your body will continue to anticipate food at breakfast time for a few days, but it will soon adapt to your new pattern. By sticking to a consistent fasting routine, it is possible that participants experienced less hunger during their fasting periods, which translated into a more sensible diet during their eating window and the observed natural decrease of calories over time.

It is also worth noting that recognizing hunger is a skill many of us have lost. The refined foods that make up so much of the standard American diet get digested and absorbed quickly into the bloodstream. The resulting blood sugar spike is followed by an inevitable crash that brings hunger back sooner than expected. On top of that, years of eating these low-value foods have left many of us insulin resistant, which means that even if we take in a lot of quick-digesting calories, our cells resist the energy and our cravings for more food never go away. With these circumstances in place, you may find it beneficial to monitor your food intake as your body relearns how to tell you when enough is enough. Until you have remastered that skill, it's a good idea to calculate your caloric needs and track your nutrient intake.

The number of calories you need depends on many factors, including your age, gender, height, current weight, activity level, and metabolic health. The easiest way to determine how many calories your body needs is to find an online calorie calculator. Although these generic calculators can't account for all of the nuances of your metabolic rate, they can get you in the ballpark. With that number in mind, you can further use technology to record your daily food and beverage intake and track your calorie and nutrient consumption using a food journaling app.

PUTTING IT ALL TOGETHER

Here are the characteristics of a healthy low-carb, high-fat diet:

1. **Carbs:** Limit your carb intake to no more than 25 percent of your total daily calories. If you choose to follow a keto diet, limit your intake to less than 10 percent. Eliminate sugar and refined carbohydrates.

2. **Fat:** Boost your fat intake to at least 50 percent of your daily calories. Choose mostly natural fats from whole foods, and avoid vegetable oils.

3. **Protein:** Take in a sufficient amount of protein equivalent to about 15 to 25 percent of your daily calories. Increase your protein intake if you're older, fighting an illness, or actively working to build muscle.

HOW TO BREAK A FAST

You now know how to eat during your eating window, but what about the transition from fasting to eating? Is there a best practice for ending a fast? The answer depends on the length of your fast. For time-restricted eating patterns in which you are eating every day, you can break your fast with a regular meal. If you have been fasting for 24 hours or more or for consecutive days, you'll do best if you reintroduce food slowly to avoid digestive issues or the rare but serious refeeding syndrome. Here are some tips to follow:

1. Make your first meal small.

2. Good choices to break a fast include bone broth, a smoothie with a bit of protein powder, or a small portion of cooked vegetables that you chew thoroughly.

3. If you feel fine after 30 to 60 minutes, consume a more substantial (but still small) meal with foods that you're used to eating.

If your goal includes better health or weight loss, the foods you choose to eat during your eating window matter. But what, if anything, can you eat or drink during your fast? You can have coffee—right? What about cream in your coffee? Is there more to learn about timing your fast and exercising in a fasted state? It's time to dig into the ins and outs of fasting.

7

THE INS + OUTS OF FASTING

What lies ahead

- **To avoid breaking your fast during your fasting window, it's best to avoid caloric foods and drinks and artificial sweeteners.** Noncaloric beverages, such as water, coffee, and tea, are okay to consume.

- **You can exercise in a fasted state, but monitor how you feel and note that your performance may be affected.** Aerobic exercise during a fast may enhance fat burning.

- **There are a variety of ways to troubleshoot if you hit a weight-loss plateau.** Sometimes, it can be helpful to throw your body a curveball with some tweaks to your diet, fasting routine, or lifestyle.

- **Take IF with you on vacations and holidays.** It's an easy way to control your weight as you enjoy life!

By this point, you have a good idea of how to eat and which fasting method will work best for you. However, as is often the case when embarking on something new, it is the subtle nuances that have the potential to trip you up. In this chapter, we'll iron out any wrinkles in your game plan so your fasting experience goes smoothly. Let's take a look at how to eat, drink, and move during your fasting window; how to handle special occasions; and what to do if you're not getting the results you expect.

WHAT BREAKS A FAST?

Before we get into what can and cannot be consumed during your fasting window, we need to define what it means to "break a fast." In the strictest sense, a fast is performed without food, drink, or substances that challenge your metabolism—in other words, water only. However, adhering to inflexible rules like this can leave you feeling uncomfortable and hungry, which jeopardizes your long-term fasting success. So is there a compromise? Are there foods or beverages that you can consume while fasting and still reap the benefits of fasting? With little research to lean on, the answer involves a fair amount of speculation. However, we can glean some insights by contemplating why fasting is so beneficial to your body. We know that going without food for long periods frees up healing resources and

allows insulin to drop to a low level. This low insulin level creates an internal environment that favors fat burning. You want to keep your body in this fat-burning mode as long as possible, so consuming something that raises insulin would work against that goal. With this understanding, let's look at common foods and beverages that you may wish to consume during your fasting period.

Water

It is wise to stay hydrated during your fast by consuming water. With no calories and no nutrients to influence your metabolism, water is a safe beverage to drink at any time during your day. You can pour yourself a glass of water from the tap or choose unsweetened mineral water or bubbly water such as carbonated water, sparkling water, club soda, or seltzer. These water options mix things up a bit and add an element of fun and satisfaction to your fast.

What if you enjoy a bit of flavor in your water? For instance, many people like to drop a slice of lemon in their glass. Lemon is a fruit, so it contains calories that will be added to the water. However, is a squeeze of lemon a deal-breaker? Although the fasting purist can argue that any calories break a fast, it is doubtful that a small amount of lemon juice is enough to destroy the benefits gained over hours of fasting. However, water sweetened with a noncaloric sweetener may be a different story.

Noncaloric Sweeteners

With no calories to speak of, you would think that sugar substitutes would be fine to use during your fasting window. Unfortunately, there is evidence that noncaloric sweeteners are not the metabolic free ride that they are made out to be. Some of them have a glycemic index, which means that they cause a rise in your blood sugar. Studies have linked these substances to altered gut health, glucose intolerance, and insulin resistance, which are all issues that can impact your ability to lose weight.[1, 2]

Here is something else to consider: there is a phenomenon referred to as the *cephalic phase insulin response*. The term *cephalic* refers to your head, so in its simplest translation, this is an insulin response that is all in your head and has nothing to do with glucose in your blood. What causes this response is merely having something sweet in your mouth. Interesting studies have been conducted that asked participants to swish different non-caloric sweetened solutions around in their mouth and then spit them out. They did not swallow the solutions, yet when their blood was drawn after the taste sensation, insulin concentrations were elevated.[3, 4] In other words, the study participants experienced a rise in their blood insulin levels even though they spit the sweet solution out of their mouths. Yikes, right? The takeaway from these studies is that "sugar-free" does not mean "care-free." These substances have an impact on your brain, body, and metabolism.

It can be argued that not all noncaloric sweeteners are created equal. I would concur that stevia and others that are derived from natural substances are better options than artificial sweeteners, like aspartame, which is used in many diet sodas. However, beyond the debate over their health value, there is one overarching reason why I recommend reducing or eliminating all sugar substitutes from your diet. Plainly stated, their intense sweetness keeps your addiction to sweets alive. Do you want that? Sugar-free foods and beverages are still sweet. So, if you continually consume them, you continually feed your sweet tooth.

The 411 on sugar substitutes

It's best to wean yourself off of all sugar substitutes. However, if desired, here are the okay (and not okay) choices:

Least-harmful sugar substitutes:

* Allulose
* Erythritol
* Monk fruit
* Pure stevia
* Swerve (a blend of erythritol and oligo-saccharides)
* Truvia (a blend of erythritol and stevia)
* Xylitol

Sugar substitutes to avoid:

* Aspartame found in Equal (blue packets) and diet soda
* Maltitol*
* Saccharin found in Sweet'N Low (pink packets)
* Sorbitol*
* Sucralose found in Splenda (yellow packets)

* Maltitol and sorbitol are sugar alcohols that are often added to gum and hard candies. These artificial sweeteners may cause stomach upset in sensitive individuals.

This is a problem because sweetness has a powerful mental and physical pull. When you constantly have sweet things on your tongue, your taste buds and brain chemistry continue to desire sweetness, and you stay hooked. Bottom line, if you need to use sugar substitutes as a crutch to get sugar out of your diet, that's fine, but you'll be happiest with your overall results if you wean yourself off of them as you progress.

Coffee and Tea

Coffee and tea may start your "metabolic clock" but are generally accepted as okay to consume during a fast. One of the advantages of IF is that it allows you to work with your body's natural metabolic rhythm by consuming food during the hours of the day when your metabolism is most active. An important activator of your metabolic clock is your first bite or sip of food or drink for the day. When your clock starts and your metabolic engine begins to rev up, your body experiences a peak in insulin sensitivity and fatty acid oxidation that gradually diminishes as the day goes on. What that means is that your body can use and process food better at the beginning of your eating window than at the end. With this understanding, you could argue that the noncaloric nutrients you ingest when you drink a cup of coffee or tea break your fast and should be avoided. However, many people would sooner jump off a cliff than give up their morning cup of joe, so let's build some arguments in support of coffee and its close relative, tea.

Why coffee and tea are okay to consume during a fast:

- Coffee makes life worth living (or at least more enjoyable).

- Many IF studies have allowed participants to consume noncaloric drinks like coffee and tea. The consumption of these drinks did not hinder their results in a significant way.

- Coffee and tea are rich in antioxidants and other helpful components that have been shown in mice studies to induce the cellular cleanup process called autophagy.[5, 6]

- We know from studies with human participants that caffeine helps your body break down fat.[7]

So there appears to be a trade-off. Your cup of coffee or tea might start your metabolic clock, which technically opens your eating window. However, if that is the only thing that you are consuming in the morning hours, you may be gaining an advantage with respect to autophagy and fat release. This leads to the next logical question, which is what, if anything, can you put in your cup?

Cream and Other Fat Calories

If a plain cup of black coffee or tea doesn't thrill you, you're likely looking to stir in a bit of flavor in the form of a fat, a sweetener, or a spice. Foods that consist mostly of fat have little impact on your blood sugar and insulin level, so consuming fat calories during your fasting period will not knock your body out of fat-burning mode. That's a good thing and the reason why most people find that they can enjoy a bit of cream or similar items in their coffee or tea without noticeable consequences.

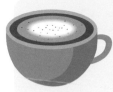

Is coffee healthy or not?

Nearly two-thirds of us start our day with a cup of coffee. Is this morning ritual okay, or are we doing our bodies harm by drinking cup after cup, day after day? As it turns out, there are good and bad sides to coffee.

Benefits:

* **Comes from the coffee bean:** When you brew a cup, the beneficial nutrients of the beans, including cell-defending antioxidants, are transferred into your cup.

* **May help you live longer:** A study published in 2012 evaluated the coffee consumption of hundreds of thousands of men and women over the age of 50 and found that "coffee consumption was inversely associated with total and cause-specific mortality."[8]

* **May protect you from diabetes:** A systematic review of the scientific literature showed "high intakes of coffee, decaffeinated coffee, and tea are associated with reduced risk of diabetes."[9]

* **Regular consumption supports fat loss:** It could be that the nutrients in the coffee combine with the metabolic boost that you get from the caffeine to give you the fat-burning advantage.[10]

* **May boost autophagy:** Although the only research to date has been done on mice, there is hope that the nutrients in coffee enhance autophagy in humans.[5, 6]

* **Makes you more alert in the short and long term:** A systematic review published in 2016 showed that "higher coffee consumption is associated with reduced risk for Alzheimer's disease."[11]

Drawbacks:

* **Can leave sensitive individuals feeling jittery:** It may also worsen feelings of anxiety.

* **Can disrupt sleep if you drink it in the afternoon:** Caffeine has a half-life of about 6 hours, which means that 6 hours after you drink a cup of coffee, half of the caffeine from that cup is still in your system. In other words, much of the caffeine from that cup you drank at 3pm is still in your system as you prepare for bed.

* **Is addictive:** If you stop drinking it, you will likely suffer withdrawal symptoms, including headaches, irritability, and brain fog.

* **Caffeine may raise your blood pressure:** More research needs to be conducted on this.[12]

* **May worsen heartburn:** Caffeine relaxes the lower esophageal sphincter, which is the barrier that keeps stomach acid from moving back up toward your throat.

However, fat has calories, and calories are energy. Your body will use those easily accessed calories before returning to the less-accessible calories stored in your fat cells. If you have three cups of coffee over the course of a morning and you add cream to each of those cups, then you are providing your body with a consistent source of energy instead of burning it from your body stores. The same can be said for keto or bulletproof coffee concoctions in which multiple fats (e.g., MCT oil, coconut oil, butter, cream, etc.) are added to a single cup of coffee. The more fat that is added, the more energy you supply to your body. Milk (including plant-based milk such as hemp or almond milk) contains a mix of fat, protein, and carbohydrates, which gives it more potential to break a fast. If milk is your preferred add-in, you'll be happiest with your results if you use full-fat milk or half-and-half.

Coffee Sweeteners and Spices

As mentioned earlier, noncaloric sweeteners can have an unexpected impact on your metabolism and health. If you cannot live without a sweetener in your coffee or tea, you'll do best with one that comes from a natural source, such as stevia or monk fruit. Honey and agave nectar are also from natural sources, but they get their sweetness from fructose, which is a type of sugar that must be metabolized by your liver, interrupting your fast. Spices, on the other hand, are used in small amounts and provide benefits for your body, so feel free to add a shake of turmeric, cinnamon, nutmeg, or other favorites to your morning brew.

Fast fact: what is MCT oil?

MCT oil is a popular oil among low-carb and keto dieters because of the unique way your body handles it. MCT stands for medium-chain triglyceride, which is a type of fat. Unlike most dietary fats, MCTs are taken directly to your liver, where they can be burned immediately for energy or turned into the alternative energy source—ketones (see page 44). Because they are directly turned into energy, there's little left over to get stored as body fat.

Although not best for cooking, MCT oil can be mixed into salad dressing or stirred into coffee or tea to help stave off hunger. It does have a laxative effect, so if you try it, start slow. I recommend starting with a teaspoon of oil a day to see how your body tolerates it. If you feel good, you can increase the amount to a tablespoon.

If you choose to use MCT powder instead of MCT oil, check the label for additives. Ingredients are often added to the powders to improve flavor and prevent clumping. These additives could impact your metabolism and potentially break your fast.

Coffee add-ins during your fast

Anything other than water has the potential to impact your fast. If you enjoy something in your coffee or tea, here's a list of items that will have the least impact:

Add this:

* Butter
* Coconut oil
* Cream (heavy cream or coconut cream)
* Full-fat milk
* Half-and-half
* MCT oil
* Spices
* Stevia or monk fruit

Not this:

* Agave nectar
* Artificial sweeteners (Equal, Splenda, Sweet'N Low)
* Honey
* Low-fat or skim milk
* Nut milk (e.g., hemp, almond, cashew, etc.)
* Sugar

SUPPLEMENTS

Whether you are aiming for a specific bodybuilding goal or looking to support a particular facet of your health, there's a supplement for that. As a general rule, the best advice on timing your supplement intake is "when in doubt, take it with food." However, this simple instruction invites a lot of "but, what if"s: "But what if I fast for longer than a day?" "But what if I need to take the supplement with a workout, before bed, or first thing in the morning?" With so many supplements on the market, it would be impossible to review all of them. However, we can group supplements together and consider how your body uses them to make educated decisions about whether to take the supplement during your eating or fasting window.

Bodybuilding and Protein Supplements

To build muscle, you need protein. If you work out during your eating window, protein is provided through your diet. However, what if you work out during your fasting window? Would taking a supplement such as whey protein or BCAAs (branched-chain amino acids) break your fast? The answer is yes, but the full question to contemplate is whether that temporary break is defeating your goal. When you fast, specific growth pathways, such as IGF-1 and mTOR, are deactivated. This is not necessarily a bad thing because these pathways must be deactivated for autophagy to happen. If your goal is to gain muscle, you want these growth pathways to be active. One way to do that is to take in amino acids. So the decision of whether or not to take a protein-based supplement during your fast comes down to how you answer this question: "Will this temporary disruption of my fast be worth the muscle growth that I stand to gain?"

Vitamins, Omega-3s, Probiotics, and Electrolytes

There are many types of supplements that you can take to support your general health. Most will be best taken with food, but if you are doing an extended fast or prefer taking them in the morning or before bed, they will still provide benefits. Let's consider a few of the more common ones:

- **Multivitamins and other fat-soluble vitamin supplements** are best taken with food to support the absorption of the fat-soluble vitamins (A, D, E, and K).

- **Water-soluble vitamin supplements** (B and C) are okay to take any time of day, whether during your fasting window or not.

- **Omega-3 fatty acids** are often consumed in capsule or liquid form, much like a vitamin. Taking them with food aids in their absorption.

- **Probiotics** are a bit tricky to figure out. They contain live microorganisms that support the beneficial bacteria living in your gut (intestines). To get down to your gut, the microorganisms must survive a long journey through your digestive tract. Whether they survive better traveling with or without food is debated, and research findings are inconclusive. So this is one of those times that our adage "when in doubt, take it with food" comes in handy.

- **Electrolytes** are essential minerals that your body needs to perform countless functions, from regulating nerve and muscle actions to keeping you hydrated.

Your body naturally loses electrolytes when fasting, so you'll need to replenish them to feel your best and avoid common issues like muscle cramps, headaches, and sleep problems. Look for an electrolyte supplement with potassium, magnesium, sodium, and chloride, and take it daily in a fasted or fed state.

Bone Broth

Bone broth is rich in amino acids, which can disrupt your fast. However, this is another instance when the benefits might outweigh the drawbacks. If you are just getting started and feeling fatigued or hungry, bone broth can support you as you work toward becoming more comfortable with fasting. If you are doing an extended fast, you may find that bone broth helps you to control hunger and feel good while preserving the overall benefits of the fast. It may also help to protect muscle mass during a prolonged fast thanks to its high protein content.

Apple Cider Vinegar

Apple cider vinegar (ACV) has been touted as a natural remedy for everything from better health to weight loss, and there is scientific evidence to support many of these claims. One study showed that taking 2 tablespoons (30ml) of ACV before a meal helped muscles to absorb the glucose from the meal.[13] Another study showed that diabetic patients who consumed 2 tablespoons of apple cider vinegar with 1 ounce of cheese (to make the vinegar more palatable) at bedtime had a reduction in their fasting blood glucose reading the next morning.[14] Because of its many benefits and the fact that it is free of calories, ACV is fine to take during your

Taking supplements while fasting

Some supplements are best absorbed when taken with food. Others have the potential to break your fast, but they provide your body with benefits that make them worthwhile to consume as you fast. Here are some general guidelines for timing your supplement intake:

Best taken during your eating window:

* BCAAs
* Bone broth
* Fat-soluble vitamins (A, D, E, and K) and multivitamins
* Fiber supplements
* Omega-3s
* Probiotics
* Whey protein and protein powders

Okay to take during your fast:

* Apple cider vinegar
* Electrolytes
* Water-soluble vitamins (B and C)

Medications: Some medications are best taken with food to ensure proper absorption. Others must be taken first thing in the morning or right before bed. Talk with your doctor about how to best take your medication while fasting.

fasting window or right before a meal. Some people also claim that taking it during their fast helps to control hunger. One note of caution: it is not the most pleasant-tasting substance, and its acidic nature can damage your throat or teeth if taken straight. By diluting a couple of tablespoons in a glass of water with lemon, you'll help the "medicine" go down.

EXERCISING WHILE FASTING

It is okay to exercise while you fast, but how you go about it will depend on your goals and how you feel. Countless health benefits come from exercise, but for many of us, the goals we seek when we embark on an exercise routine are to build muscle or lose fat. In Chapter 5, you learned that it is possible to maintain and even build muscle while practicing IF. However, because studies on muscle growth and fasting had participants work out during their eating window and

consume whey protein soon after exercising, it remains unclear if the same muscle-building benefits can be reaped if you work out during your fast. My personal experience says that you can still build muscle in a fasted state, but the jury is still out on that one.

Fasting cyclist

"I'm a 62-year-old cyclist and I'm post-menopause for a decade. I wanted to lose a pesky 9lbs. IF has helped me lose 6lbs over the course of 6 weeks. I've been keeping to about 1,600 calories during breakfast and lunch, and then fasting till the next breakfast. Doing 16:8, I notice a significant decrease in muscle and joint soreness in the morning and increased aerobic capacity during my workouts."

—Missy P.

However, what about specifically performing aerobic exercise in the fasted state? What if you wake up, shake off the sleepiness, and head over to the gym for an hour of cardio, or slip outside for a brisk morning walk or jog around the neighborhood? The goal of aerobic exercise is not to build the body, but rather to burn calories and increase overall fitness. In this case, the research is clear that aerobic training in a fasted state has many perks, including better fat burning and energy uptake by your cells.

- A study published in 2016 analyzed the findings from previous research and found that aerobic exercise performed in the fasted state enhanced fat burning compared to exercise done in the fed state.[15]

- A 6-week study had healthy men perform four 60- to 90-minute exercise sessions per week. Some of the men ate before and during the exercise session while others exercised in a fasted state. Those who exercised without food were more efficient at using energy and burning fat.[16]

- A study that involved 30 overweight or obese men showed that engaging in moderately intense aerobic exercise before eating breakfast doubled their fat burning compared to when they ate breakfast before their workout.[17]

Fasted exercise

"IF took me a long time to get used to, but almost right away I noticed that fasted exercise was amazing. I normally exercise in the morning at the 16-or-so-hour fast marker, and it is great. A few times, I've scheduled tennis to start at my eating time. Instead of eating, I played first, and it's the best energy I have had."

—Lance L.

Fast fact: feel-good fasting tips

Your body is a marvelous machine that can adapt to almost anything you throw at it. But it is also somewhat of a stubborn old coot that is set in its ways, meaning that when you throw something new at it, like fasting, it puts up a fuss for a few days. For many people, this uncomfortable feeling will pass on its own as your body adapts to your new routine, but there are some general ways to support your body as you fast that will improve how you feel:

* **Drink water.** There is a form of fasting referred to as "dry fasting" in which a person abstains from all food and drink, including water. Proponents claim that this complete form of fasting boosts weight loss, improves immune function, and reduces inflammation. However, the evidence to support these claims is not strong, and going without water could be dangerous and lead to increased hunger, fatigue, brain fog, irritability, and headaches. Bottom line: drink plenty of water during both your fasting and eating windows.

* **Add an electrolyte or mineral supplement.** When you fast, you lower your insulin level and deplete glycogen stores that hold water in your body. This depletion of glycogen and water is amplified if you pair your fast with a low-carb diet. As the water leaves your body, electrolytes tag along. Electrolytes are minerals that carry an electric charge when immersed in the watery environments of your body. Certain electrolytes like magnesium, potassium, sodium, and chloride regulate vital processes, from fluid balance to nerve and muscle function. If your body is running low, you may feel tired and moody and experience muscle cramps and trouble sleeping. Fortunately, there are many easy ways to take in these substances:

    * Add a pinch of sea salt to your food or drink to get sodium, chloride, and other trace minerals.

    * Take a daily multivitamin or electrolyte supplement.

    * Drink bone broth, which is rich in minerals and other micronutrients.

    * Add Epsom salt to your bath of warm water. Although it's debated how much of the magnesium in Epsom salt can be absorbed through the skin, the warm soak will calm muscle soreness and cramping.

* **Avoid too much, too soon.** When motivation strikes, it's tempting to change everything at once. You proclaim that today is the day, so you begin fasting, overhaul your diet, and join a gym. Although it may be true that multiple aspects of your health could use some improvement, tackling them all at once will leave you feeling drained and make you prone to quit. Instead, take a round-one, round-two approach:

Round one:

* Start with a 12-hour fast, and work up to 14 hours.

* Continue with your typical exercise routine, or add a light exercise like walking.

* Don't focus on cutting calories until hunger is under control.

* Follow the basic 0–1–2–3 rules to get your diet on track.

* Add cream or another fat to your coffee to control hunger.

Round two:

* Follow a 16-hour fast, or try an alternate-day routine.

* Boost your exercise time and intensity.

* Determine your calorie limit, and start tracking your food intake.

* Reduce your carbohydrate intake to accelerate weight loss.

* Try a water-only fast.

It is clear that IF can help you sculpt the body you want, but will exercise in the fasted state impact how you feel or perform? The answer to this question is somewhat subjective because some people feel better working out on an empty stomach, whereas others feel like they need a little gas in the tank to perform their best at the gym. The research on exercise performance and fasting is also divided and may depend on your starting fitness level. A study done on elite judo athletes who fasted during Ramadan found that, despite increased fatigue, their athletic performance did not suffer significantly.[18] Studies on endurance athletes also showed that they maintained their performance level when training in a fasted state.[19] However, research on untrained athletes revealed a mixed bag of results. Some studies showed no change in performance, while others reported improved or impaired performance.[20]

The bottom line is that physical training and fasting can work together and have beneficial effects on your body composition, insulin sensitivity, and overall health. However, if you exercise in a fasted state, you should monitor how you feel and stop if you are feeling light-headed or unwell.

WHAT IF YOU DON'T FEEL WELL?

It's discouraging when you set out to improve your health and end up feeling worse rather than better. Although this dip in how you feel is often temporary, it can cause you to throw in the towel before the magic happens. There is a line that must be drawn between feeling a touch under the weather and facing

a serious health threat. As a rule, it's best to err on the side of caution and connect with your doctor about any symptoms that do not feel right to you. However, feeling a bit out of sorts or experiencing an uptick in fatigue, cravings, headaches, and discomfort are common symptoms anytime you change the way you feed or move your body. Let's consider some symptoms that you might encounter as you begin or continue to fast and what to do to feel better.

Hunger and Cravings

Hunger is a fickle thing. It will rise and fall throughout your day based on hormone and blood sugar levels as well as environmental cues. Smell fresh-baked bread...become instantly hungry for fresh-baked bread. Because of its come-and-go nature, you can expect to experience twinges of hunger during your fasting hours, but you can also count on them to subside. In other words, you don't need to feed hunger to satisfy hunger. A craving is a similar creature. We all get cravings when we are faced with the candy dish or the pizza commercial. Like hunger, remind yourself that this, too, shall pass. If waiting it out is not enough, try using a stopper (see page 86). Of course, that doesn't mean that hunger and cravings are fun to experience. Here are some practical ways to quiet them.

The fixes:

- **Ride out hunger.** Your body learns your habits and patterns. When you skip a typical meal, your body reminds you to eat by stimulating your appetite. Work on riding out the hunger wave, and within a few days, your body will learn your new fasting routine, and hunger will diminish naturally.

- **Eat enough.** It's common to want to push the limits and try to speed up fat loss by drastically cutting calories. However, this strategy can backfire, sparking your hunger and slowing your metabolism.

- **Eat fat.** It's tempting to cut fats out of your diet because these foods are very calorie-dense. If you cut out nuts, seeds, avocados, and other high-fat foods, thinking you'll save a few calories, what you are really doing is inviting hunger.

- **Sleep.** Being sleep deprived alters your hunger hormones, leaving you feeling hungrier than usual throughout the day. Darken your bedroom as much as possible, lower the room temperature, and aim for 7 to 9 hours of restful sleep.

Muscle Cramps

Muscles seem pretty straightforward. They are what take us on a stroll, lift a bag of groceries, and raise the glass to our lips. At least that's what we see on the surface. Inside, each muscle contraction requires a complex interplay between the muscle fibers and your nervous system, and this entire dance is reliant on minerals, particularly magnesium, calcium, sodium, and potassium. If these minerals are lacking, the muscles seize up, leaving you with a cramp that stops you in your tracks or springs you out of bed. Because fasting causes water and electrolytes to flush out of the body more readily, it's not uncommon to experience cramps and spasms. The good news is that when nutrient deficiencies cause them, they are corrected with nutrient intake.

The fixes:

- **Add electrolytes.** You can pick up an electrolyte supplement at your local pharmacy or online.

- **Drink mineral water.** Mineral water comes from a mineral spring and contains a host of trace minerals that can ward off muscle cramps.

- **Eat magnesium-rich foods.** I refer to magnesium as "mellow magnesium" because it has a wide range of calming effects on your body, from more relaxed muscles to less anxiety. A properly prepared daily salad is one of the best vehicles for filling your body with magnesium-rich foods! (A bed of dark leafy greens along with pumpkin seeds, slivered almonds, and slices of avocado gives you a good dose of magnesium and makes for a great-tasting salad.)

Constipation

For some people, it's a simple matter of quantity. With less food coming in, there is less waste going out. This lower volume can be mistaken for constipation. That being said, any change to your diet can result in changes in bowel movements. If you experience constipation while fasting, you can take steps to get things moving. However, keep in mind that there are many reasons for constipation. If these natural remedies don't work, discuss the matter with your doctor.

The fixes:

- **Stay hydrated.** Drink plenty of water (at least 8 glasses/day), and supplement your diet with electrolytes. You'll maintain water balance in your body, which helps stool pass more easily.

- **Add fiber.** Your fiber intake may have dropped when you started fasting or reduced your carb intake. Not everyone experiences constipation relief with added fiber, but you might find it does the trick.

  - Psyllium husk is the active ingredient in Metamucil, which is an over-the-counter constipation aid. Look for organic psyllium husk to avoid pesticides and additives.

  - Chia seeds are high in fiber and can absorb water, which helps soften stool. Because of their mild taste, they are an easy addition to yogurt and smoothies.

  - Add vegetables with a high fiber-to-carb ratio, such as dark leafy greens, asparagus, cauliflower, and sauerkraut.

- **Add MCT oil.** This unique oil has a laxative effect. Start with a teaspoon of MCT oil stirred into your coffee or tea, and work up to a tablespoon per day.

- **Add exercise.** Movement of the bowels relies somewhat on muscular contractions, so if you have a history of constipation, you may want to work on improving your core muscle strength through exercise. Although walking does not significantly improve core strength, it can help with motility, so a brisk walk once or twice a day may be beneficial.

Tiredness, Mental Fog, and Irritability

When you change your eating routine, your body needs a few days to adjust, during which time you may feel sluggish, moody, and mentally foggy. However, before long, the fog should lift and you should experience a heightened and sustained level of energy and well-being. Here are some things that will help your body ease into fasting without the consequences or give your body a pick-me-up as you continue on your fasting routine.

The fixes:

- **Start with a 12:12 fast.** A 12-hour fast that's performed overnight allows your body and mind time to adapt to going without food. When you're comfortable, stretch your fasting period to 14 or 16 hours.

- **Add as you subtract.** As you reduce the number of hours you eat, you'll want to add micronutrients to avoid dehydration and deficiencies. Easy ways to do this are to add a multivitamin, electrolyte supplement, mineral water, or bone broth.

- **Eat enough protein.** Most people will do fine with a moderate protein intake in which 15 to 25 percent of their daily calories come from protein. However, if you are feeling sluggish, you may find that you feel best when you keep your protein intake at or above 25 percent.

- **Ditch the empty calories.** If you feel like your energy tank is empty, then it's time to ditch the empty calories found in processed and refined foods.

Severe Fatigue, Dizziness, Light-Headedness, Confusion, Shakiness, and Nausea

Severe fatigue, nausea, confusion, and any other debilitating sensations are not normal side effects of fasting. If you experience any of these symptoms, you should stop fasting immediately and contact your doctor.

WHAT IF YOU'RE NOT LOSING WEIGHT?

You've been fasting routinely and eating a decent diet, so you expect to see results, but when you step on the scale, the results aren't there. What's going on? Although it's not uncommon to experience a temporary stall in weight loss, hitting a full-blown plateau is never fun. Let's take a look at some things that can impact weight loss and ways to get the scale moving down:

- **Check your medications.** Several medications can slow weight loss, including but not limited to antidepressants, antihistamines, birth control, statins, and steroid anti-inflammatories, as well as medications for blood pressure, diabetes, and migraines. If you are taking a prescribed drug and having trouble losing weight, ask your doctor if there is a connection.

- **Keep going.** A plateau that lasts for a couple of weeks does not necessarily indicate that something is wrong with your plan. Your body is a complex and intelligent machine, and try as you might, its actions are often hard to predict. Sometimes, instead of a forceful hand, all it needs is time. Although steady and consistent effort may be the boring path, it is often the strategy that wins in the long run.

- **Clean up your diet.** Fasting can mitigate some of the adverse health effects of a poor diet. However, if your eating window is filled with refined carbs (e.g., bread, energy bars, pasta, and sweetened drinks or soda), you may be blocking weight loss by elevating your insulin level and taking in too many calories. Check out the recipes and meal plans provided in Part 2, and use them as a guide to healthy eating.

- **Reduce your carbs.** Low-carb diets work because they rob your body of the easy-to-burn carbohydrates, forcing it to burn fat for fuel. If your weight loss has stalled, reduce your carb intake. If you already follow a low-carb diet, watch out for hidden carbs and "carb creep," which is the tendency for additional carbs to sneak into your diet as you progress toward your goal. ("A small cookie shouldn't matter.") Take a few days to read labels and track how many grams of carbs you're actually taking in and then reduce the number until the scale is moving again.

- **Change your fasting method.** One of the best ways to shake a plateau is to throw your body a curveball. Your body is always looking for ways to conserve energy, so it quickly learns your new pattern and becomes efficient, which requires less energy and fewer calories. If your weight loss has stalled, mix things up by adding a longer fast once or twice a week or cycling calorie intake with a modified alternate-day routine.

- **Lengthen your fast.** Everyone's metabolism is different. Although a 16-hour fast might work wonders for your friend, you might not see results until you've fasted for 20 hours.

- **Fast early rather than late.** In the evening hours, your circadian clock influences the production of hormones that prepare you for sleep. Eating too close to bedtime can work against this hormonal shift, keeping your blood sugar elevated and blocking fat burning overnight. To encourage weight loss, stop eating a minimum of 3 hours before bed, and eat the majority of calories at the beginning of your eating window.

- **Change your eating frequency.** It's true that eating gives your metabolic rate a boost. However, this increase is minimal and countered by the resulting increase in insulin that can block fat release. To change things up, try eating two meals during your eating window rather than three.

- **Move more.** Exercise improves insulin sensitivity, which is a mark of how well your cells take in and use energy. We all have a unique starting point when it comes to exercise. If you've been inactive, focus on increasing your physical activity with fun activities like walking or gardening. If you are currently active, try increasing the intensity or length of your workouts.

FASTING STRATEGIES FOR SPECIAL OCCASIONS

Intermittent fasting is a weight-control strategy that you can follow all year long, even during the times that you take a break from your normal routine, like holidays and vacations. These special, treat-filled moments entice many of us to put a hold on self-control and eat with abandon. This mindset is human nature, and being human myself, I don't begrudge anyone for taking a few days off to break the rules. However, these occasional days of indulgence can add up, contributing to the 1 to 2 pounds of weight the average person puts on each year. At least that's how it used to be. Now you have a secret weapon, intermittent fasting, that you can use to turn around a short-lived sidestep before it becomes permanent weight gain. Here are some tricks I rely on to enjoy life's celebrations without losing ground.

Fasting During the Holidays

There is no question that the holidays bring many opportunities to overeat. From the mashed potatoes to the bread stuffing to the cookie exchange, big meals and holiday snacks tend to be very heavy in carbs. Not only do these foods raise insulin, they also cause your body to retain water, making the scale a scary thing to confront the day after a celebration. Fortunately, fasting after a feast accelerates the elimination of excess water and stabilizes insulin. Fasting should never be looked at as punishment for overindulging; instead, look at it as the ace up your sleeve that gives you the upper hand

and puts you back in control. To get back on track quickly, try lengthening your fasting window the next day or two after a feast. For instance, if you typically fast for 16 hours, try a 20-hour fast or OMAD after a holiday meal. You can also take a proactive step by making the holiday meal your only meal of the day.

Fasting on Vacation

When I travel, I've found that spreading out my eating and having the right mindset helps to prevent weight gain. On vacation, I try to limit my meals to two a day. Which two meals I choose to eat will vary. For instance, if I'm staying at a hotel that offers a complimentary breakfast, I take advantage of it; eat a large, low-carb breakfast; and then wait until dinner to eat again. If it works to skip breakfast, I have lunch and dinner only for that day. As for mindset, it has the power to make you overeat or keep you on track. For instance, if you go into a vacation with the mindset that "I am on vacation, so I deserve to splurge," that's fine, but you will have a lot of work to do when you get home. However, if you go into your vacation with the mindset that "I'm leaving my options open, but I want to feel good," you give yourself some flexibility without feeling trapped by your diet. This beneficial mindset allows you to indulge in a treat or two without the coma-inducing impact of a feeding frenzy.

YOUR NEW INTERMITTENT FASTING LIFESTYLE

So, there you have it. Together, we've gone on a journey in which we questioned well-established beliefs, explored promising research, and charted a path to better health that fits into your lifestyle without taking over your life. At times, you likely felt challenged; at others, hopeful and empowered. Admittedly, putting IF into action requires a paradigm shift, but it's not long into this new practice that the results prove worth the effort. It's a true accelerator of health, weight loss, and well-being.

I feel blessed by the opportunity to share this easy-to-follow, enjoyable, and effective strategy with you. Fasting has been around for thousands of years, yet its newfound benefits make it feel as if a great secret has been unveiled— a secret that has the potential to reverse the madness of overly complex diets. There is so much freedom waiting for you when you put fasting into practice. If you haven't done so already, take your first step and discover for yourself how this ancient healing practice can shape your future health. Now turn the page to learn about the meal plans!

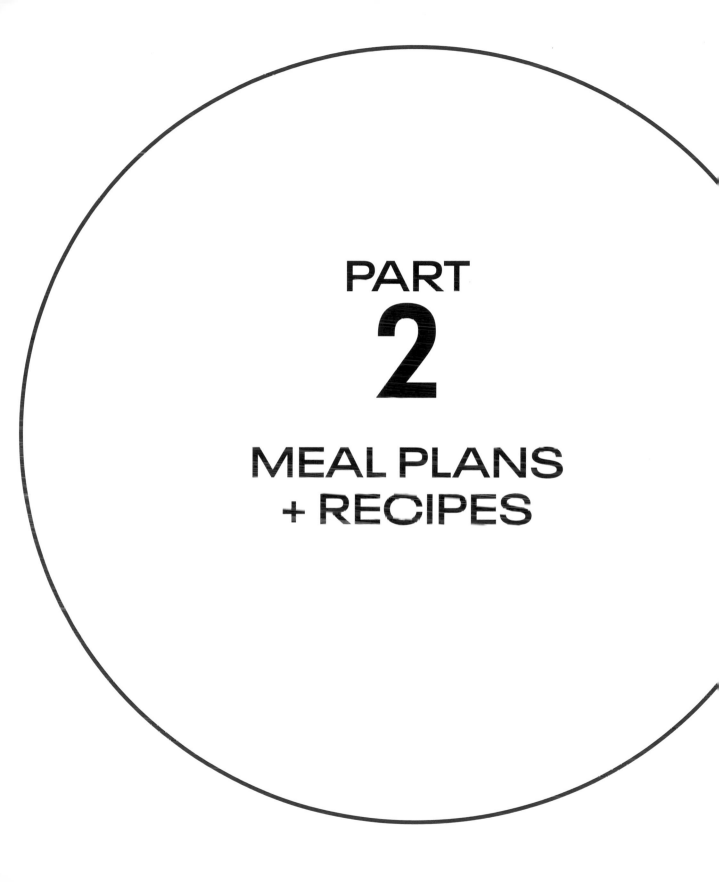

PART
2

MEAL PLANS
+ RECIPES

It's time to eat! You will maximize your fasting results by eating whole, unprocessed foods during your eating window. In this section, you'll learn which foods to choose and how to combine those foods into healthy and satisfying daily menus. The meal plans and recipes that follow show you how to eat in a way that stabilizes your blood sugar. This way of eating keeps your hunger under control and fat storage to a minimum, making for more enjoyable and effective fasting.

THE MEAL PLANS

On the following pages, you'll find made-for-you meal plans. The plans provide you with lower-carb recipes organized in a way that ensures you are getting the right mix of fat, protein, and carbs for the day. You get a full week of low-carb menus that keep your carb intake at or below 25 percent of the day's calories. You also get a full week of keto menus with 10 percent or less of the daily calories from carbs. As a bonus, you get a 3-day sample menu for those wishing to eat dairy-free or vegetarian.

To standardize the meal plans, each day's calorie count is set to about 1,400 calories, and all of the plans provide suggestions for three meals per day. It is traditional to think of these meals as breakfast, lunch, and dinner, and the recipes that follow the meal plans have been organized in a way that fits that traditional mold. However, when you practice fasting, it helps to forgo those labels and focus instead on the timing of meals during the day. Therefore, you have permission to eat eggs for dinner, break your fast at any time, or skip a meal based on your desired fasting routine.

There is no right or wrong meal plan to start with, but if you are new to low-carb dieting, I recommend starting with the low-carb meal plan. If you are an experienced low-carb dieter, you may feel comfortable jumping right into the very low-carb menus of the keto meal plan.

You have options regarding how much and how often to eat based on your hunger level. For example, if you are not feeling hungry, you can skip a meal and eat once or twice during your eating window, or if you are hungry during your eating window, then you can have all three meals or have two meals and a snack. Hunger varies based on activity level and other factors, so feel free to vary how you eat from day to day.

Adjusting Calories

Although the standard count of 1,400 calories in the meal plans will be right for some, others will need to adjust the menus to increase or decrease calories. Determining the right number of calories for you is far from an exact science. However, you can get a ballpark figure using an online calculator and then fine-tune your needs based on hunger and results on the scale. The recipes in the book offer suggestions for increasing fat or protein.

If you want to increase calorie intake:

- Add a snack that is mostly fat and protein, like a hard-boiled egg, cheese, meat, nuts, seeds, or nonstarchy veggies with guacamole or full-fat dip.

Making the meal plans work with your fasting strategy

The meal plans will help you to create a way of fasting that is all your own. Here are a few suggestions and examples to get your started.

	12:12 fast	16:8 fast	20:4 fast	OMAD	Alternate-day fast	Modified ADF
Suggestion	Eat all 3 meals within 12 hours. Add a snack if needed.	Eat 2 or 3 meals within 8 hours. Add a snack if hunger is an issue.	Choose 2 meals from the day's menu, or have 1 meal and a snack within 4 hours.	Choose 1 meal for the day and have a double portion. Add a snack if needed.	For your eating days, select the daily menus that sound the most appetizing. Add snacks if needed.	Choose any daily menus and snacks for your eating days. On fasting days, consume 500 to 600 calories.
Example	Stop eating after dinner. Delay breakfast until 12 hours have passed.	Stop eating after dinner. Skip breakfast. Resume eating at lunch.	Delay lunch until 2pm. Finish eating dinner by 6pm.	Eat 1 large meal for the day within a 1-hour window. Finish eating at least 3 hours before bed.	Eat your meals and snacks at any time on your eating days. Avoid food and caloric drinks on alternate days.	Eat as you'd like on your eating days. On fasting days, choose a meal or have a meal and a snack throughout your day.

- Add fat to your coffee or tea, such as cream or MCT oil (see pages 104–107).
- Eat an additional portion of a menu item.

If you want to decrease caloric intake:

- Avoid snacking between meals.
- Limit or avoid fat in coffee and tea.
- Reduce portion sizes.
- Eat two meals from the daily menu instead of three.

You'll be happiest with your overall results if you avoid stringing multiple low-calorie days together in a row. Although your body may handle a day or two of low-calorie intake without consequence, multiple days could result in slowing your metabolism. Here again, if you intend to go on an extended fast, do so under your doctor's supervision.

Swapping Meals in the Plan

You can rearrange or replace meals within the plans. However, keep in mind that the nutrition for each daily menu has been calculated. Therefore, you'll get the best results when you match the macronutrient breakdown of the meals you're swapping. You might find it easier to trade an entire day of eating as opposed to moving meals around. For instance, if you don't like dinner on day 4, but you enjoyed what you ate on day 1, you could eat the same menu on days 1 and 4.

Adjusting Macronutrients

Whether you're following the meal plans or creating your own, you may want to adjust certain macronutrients. Here are suggestions:

If you want to reduce carbs:

- Limit or omit fruit.

- Limit or omit starchy foods (grains, beans, corn, or potatoes).

- If you follow a keto diet, you can limit your carbs by reducing your intake of nonstarchy vegetables.

If you want to increase protein:

- Add high-protein foods, such as meat, poultry, fish, eggs, yogurt, and cheese. Plant-based options include beans, nuts, and seeds.

- Use a collagen or protein powder supplement.

If you want to increase fat:

- Add fat to your coffee or tea, such as cream or MCT oil.

- Add whole fats, such as full-fat yogurt, nuts, seeds, avocados, fatty fish, meat, eggs, and cheese.

- Cook vegetables in butter.

How to calculate macros

Because you know how many calories are in each gram of fat, protein, and carb (see page 91), you can calculate the macronutrient breakdown of your diet.

For instance, let's say you consumed 93 grams of fat, 70 grams of protein, and 70 grams of carbs. You can use the following equations to analyze your day of eating:

1. Calculate the calories per macronutrient.
Multiply the number of calories per gram by the grams eaten to get the calories per nutrient.

	Calories per gram	Grams eaten	Calories per nutrient
Fats	9	93	837
Protein	4	70	280
Carbohydrates	4	70	280
		Total daily calories = 1,397	

2. Calculate the percentage of calories per macronutrient.
By adding the total calories from each nutrient, you see that your total calorie intake for the day equals 1,397. With this information, you can determine the percentage of calories that came from each macronutrient.

Divide the calories from each nutrient by the total calories:

* 837 calories fat ÷ 1,397 calories total = **60% of calories from fat**

* 280 calories protein ÷ 1,397 calories total = **20% of calories from protein**

* 280 calories carbs ÷ 1,397 calories total = **20% of calories from carbs**

STOCKING YOUR LOW-CARB PANTRY

The following lists provide practical suggestions for adding the best sources of nutrients to your diet. You'll notice some foods appear on more than one list. For example, an egg is high in fat, but it also contains a noteworthy amount of protein. Nutrition calculators such as MyFitnessPal and Cronometer can tell you the specific nutrient breakdown of a food.

Healthy Fats

When you consume foods that are mainly fat, you do not experience a spike in blood sugar or insulin. Therefore, aim for at least 50 percent of your daily calories to come from healthy fats like the ones listed.

- Avocados
- Eggs
- Fatty fish
- Full-fat dairy
- High-quality meats
- Nuts and seeds
- Cooking fats (butter, lard, tallow)
- Cold-pressed oils (coconut oil, olive oil, avocado oil)

Healthy Proteins

A moderate intake of protein (15 to 25 percent of your daily calories) will meet the needs of the average individual. You can obtain healthy choices from both animal and plant products.

Animal proteins:
- Dairy products (cheese, milk, yogurt)
- Eggs
- Fish and seafood
- Meat (including organs) from beef, poultry, lamb, pork, and game animals

Plant proteins:
- Beans and other legumes
- Nuts and seeds
- Whole grains

Healthy Carbohydrates

Although all plant foods contain carbs, that doesn't rule them out of a healthy, low-carb diet. You just need to pick wisely so you're getting the vital nutrients from the plant foods without excess carbs. Here, you'll find lists of good low-carb plant choices.

Fruits:

Fruits are packed with nutrients, but if you have a stubborn metabolism, the natural sugars in fruit could make it hard for you to lose weight. If you have trouble losing weight, limit your fruit intake and choose fruits with the lowest net carbs.

Fruits listed from lowest to highest net carbs (net carbs based on a 3.5oz/100g serving)

- Avocados 1.8g
- Blackberries 4.3g
- Raspberries 5.4g
- Strawberries 5.7g
- Coconuts 6.2g
- Lemons 6.5g
- Watermelon 7.2g
- Cantaloupe 7.3g
- Limes 7.7g
- Peaches 8g
- Honeydew 8.3g
- Grapefruit 9.1g
- Apricots 9.1g
- Oranges 9.4g
- Plums 10g
- Apples 11.4g

- Mandarins 11.5g
- Pineapple 11.7g
- Kiwifruits 11.7g
- Pears 12g
- Blueberries 12.1g
- Mangoes 13.4g
- Cherries 13.9g
- Grapes 17.2g
- Bananas 20.2g

Vegetables:

Not all vegetables are created equal. Some contain starch, which makes them higher in carbs than their nonstarchy counterparts. Here you'll find a list of popular nonstarchy vegetables that are good choices for your low-carb lifestyle.

- Asparagus
- Broccoli
- Brussels sprouts
- Cabbage
- Cauliflower
- Celery
- Collard greens
- Cucumbers
- Eggplants
- Green beans
- Leafy greens
- Mushrooms
- Onions
- Peppers
- Sugar snap peas and snow peas
- Tomatoes
- Zucchini/summer squash

To bulk up your diet with vegetables, eat 2 cups of them either roasted in the oven, sautéed, or steamed. Adding fats, salt, and other herbs and spices makes them a tasty and healthy part of your diet. Starchy vegetables contain a high amount of carbs per serving, so you should avoid them on a keto diet and eat small amounts only on a low-carb diet. These include potatoes, starchy squashes, parsnips, green peas, and corn. Carrots fall in the middle between nonstarchy and starchy, so you'll do best if you limit the number of carrots you eat in a day.

Nuts and seeds:

Nuts and seeds can be a tasty and nutritious addition to your low-carb diet. However, be mindful of your portion size; they are easy to overeat, which could skyrocket your carb or calorie count. It's best to stick with raw versions or to roast your own nuts to avoid the unhealthy oils used in commercial roasting. Here you'll find a list of nuts and seeds that can be worked into a low-carb diet.

- Almonds
- Brazil nuts
- Chia seeds
- Flaxseeds
- Hazelnuts (a.k.a. filberts)
- Hempseeds
- Macadamia nuts
- Pecans
- Pine nuts
- Pumpkin seeds
- Sesame seeds
- Sunflower seeds
- Walnuts

Toasting nuts at home enhances the flavor. Oven-toasted nuts have the best overall color because they brown more evenly, but a skillet works, too. For amounts up to ½ cup, fry in a small pan (without any fat) over medium heat, stirring often, until golden. For amounts over ½ cup, toast the nuts on a baking sheet at 350°F (180°C) for 5 to 10 minutes or until golden brown. Store toasted nuts in airtight containers in the freezer for up to 3 months.

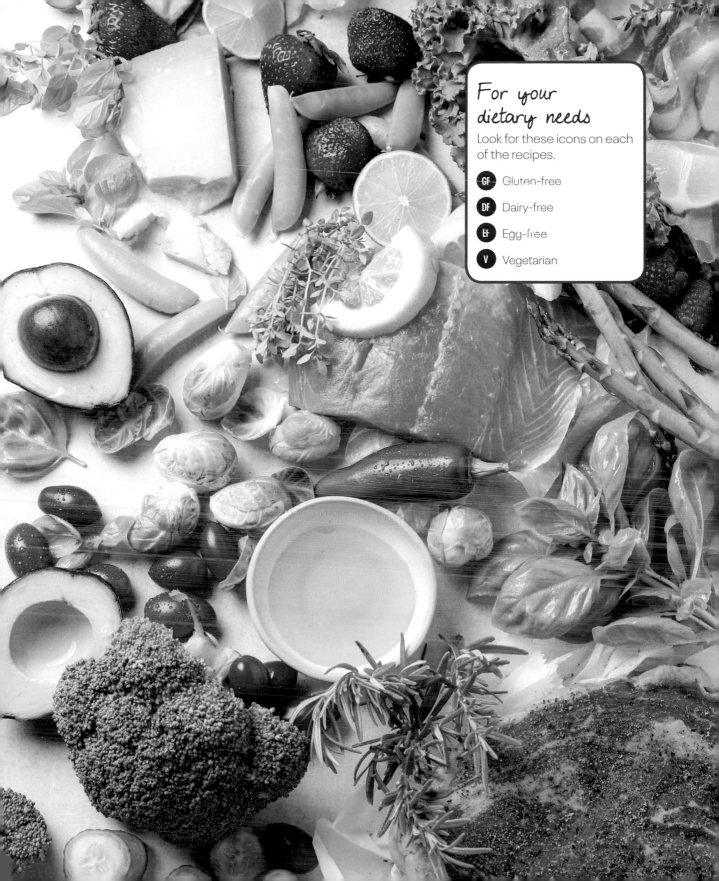

For your dietary needs

Look for these icons on each of the recipes.

GF Gluten-free

DF Dairy-free

EF Egg-free

V Vegetarian

LOW-CARB MEAL PLAN

Following this low-carb meal plan will keep insulin low, which promotes consistent fat burning. This diet is perfect for those who are new to low-carb dieting and who enjoy a variety of plant and animal foods in their diet.

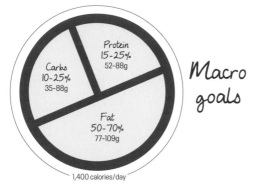

Protein
15-25%
52-88g

Carbs
10-25%
35-88g

Fat
50-70%
77-109g

Macro goals

1,400 calories/day

How to Do It

- Create a weekly shopping list, and prep food ahead of time. Have low-carb snacks ready, such as hard-boiled eggs, avocados, cheese, nuts, or nonstarchy veggies with full-fat dip.

- See page 121 for instructions specific to your fasting plan.

- You can add cream and other fats to coffee and tea, but you'll want to account for the calories.

Weekly schedule	Day 1	Day 2	Day 3
Meal 1	**Chocolate Coconut "Oats"** *p. 138* Calories 399 *Fat 33g | Carbs 19g | Protein 11g*	**Smoked Salmon with Egg and Asparagus** *p. 136* Calories 262 *Fat 19g | Carbs 12g | Protein 17g*	**Grab-and-Go Chocolate Berry Muffins** *p. 140* *(1 muffin/person)* Calories 257 *Fat 22g | Carbs 12g | Protein 6g*
Meal 2	**Grilled Green Goodness Salad** *p. 158* Calories 477 *Fat 30g | Carbs 31g | Protein 27g*	**Turkey and Avocado Asian Cabbage Salad** *p. 160* Calories 621 *Fat 46g | Carbs 29g | Protein 28g*	**Meatball Herb Salad with Olive Dressing** *p. 161* Calories 647 *Fat 49g | Carbs 33g | Protein 23g*
Meal 3	**Chicken and Broccoli Caesar Salad** *p. 162* Calories 535 *Fat 38g | Carbs 16g | Protein 36g*	**Greek Meatballs with Chunky Tomato Sauce** *p. 192* Calories 471 *Fat 33g | Carbs 17g | Protein 28g* *(make extra meatballs for day 3)* **½ cup blueberries** *(per person; eat any time of day)* Calories 42 *Fat 0g | Carbs 9g | Protein 1g*	**Shrimp Fried Cauliflower Rice** *p. 186* Calories 495 *Fat 28g | Carbs 23g | Protein 40g*
Totals	**Calories 1,411** **Fat 101g** (64%) | **Carbs 66g** (19%) *Fiber 24g* | **Protein 74g** (21%)	**Calories 1,396** **Fat 98g** (63%) | **Carbs 67g** (19%) *Fiber 20g* | **Protein 74g** (21%)	**Calories 1,399** **Fat 99g** (64%) | **Carbs 68g** (19%) *Fiber 18g* | **Protein 69g** (20%)

Greek Meatballs with Chunky Tomato Sauce (page 192)

Day 4	Day 5	Day 6	Day 7
Mushroom and Asparagus Frittata p. 151 Calories 381 *Fat 26g | Carbs 13g | Protein 32g*	**Tomato Baked Eggs** p. 146 Calories 330 *Fat 20g | Carbs 23g | Protein 16g*	**Mexican Omelet** p. 148 Calories 450 *Fat 35g | Carbs 13g | Protein 24g*	**Vanilla Cinnamon Pancakes** p. 134 Calories 384 *Fat 34g | Carbs 16g | Protein 15g*
Smoked Salmon Salad p. 157 and **Sesame Seed Bun** p. 206 (½ bun/person) Calories 504 *Fat 34g | Carbs 28g | Protein 21g*	**Chicken and Broccoli Caesar Salad** p. 162 Calories 535 *Fat 38g | Carbs 16g | Protein 36g*	**Strawberry Goat Cheese Salad with Poppy Seed Dressing** p. 164 Calories 609 *Fat 41g | Carbs 40g | Protein 10g*	**Chicken Ranch Chop Salad** p. 165 Calories 433 *Fat 27g | Carbs 12g | Protein 38g*
Mexican Meatloaf p. 184 and **Spanish Cauliflower Rice** p. 204 (2 servings/person) Calories 551 *Fat 38g | Carbs 24g | Protein 32g*	**Slow-Cooked Pork and Slaw Tacos** p. 195 Calories 464 *Fat 29g | Carbs 26g | Protein 27g*	**Roasted Herb Chicken and Gravy** p. 178 and **Cheesy Mashed Cauliflower** p. 201 (1 serving/person) and **Almond Thyme Green Beans** p. 200 (1 serving/person) Calories 377 *Fat 21g | Carbs 12g | Protein 37g*	**Creamy Mushroom Soup** p. 191 and **Garlic Rolls** p. 207 (½ roll/person) Calories 490 *Fat 37g | Carbs 26g | Protein 16g* - - - - - - - - - - - - - **1 cup blueberries** *(per person; eat any time of day)* Calories 84 *Fat 0g | Carbs 18g | Protein 2g*
Calories 1,436 **Fat 97g** (60%) | **Carbs 65g** (18%) *Fiber 22g* | **Protein 85g** (24%)	**Calories 1,329** **Fat 87g** (59%) | **Carbs 65g** (20%) *Fiber 23g* | **Protein 79g** (24%)	**Calories 1,436** **Fat 97g** (61%) | **Carbs 65g** (18%) *Fiber 18g* | **Protein 71g** (20%)	**Calories 1,391** **Fat 98g** (63%) | **Carbs 72g** (21%) *Fiber 23g* | **Protein 71g** (20%)

KETO MEAL PLAN

The menus in this meal plan keep your carbs very low, which helps your body get into ketosis to maximize fat burning. This diet is perfect for anyone who has trouble losing weight and enjoys hearty meals focused on high-fat protein choices and vegetables.

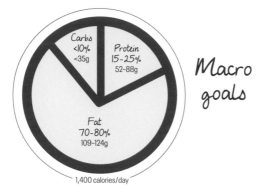

Macro goals

1,400 calories/day

How to Do It

- Create a weekly shopping list, and prep food ahead of time. Have keto snacks ready, such as hard-boiled eggs and cheese.

- See page 121 for instructions specific to your fasting plan.

- Listed nutrition facts exclude optional garnishes, so be aware that adding them could increase your daily carb count.

- It can be challenging to limit carbs while eating 2 cups nonstarchy veggies. Daily greens and veggies are reduced as needed.

- Days 4 and 6 include Keto Coffee to increase fat. See page 104 to decide when to drink the coffee. You can add cream and other fats to coffee and tea on other days, but you'll want to account for the calories.

Weekly schedule	Day 1	Day 2	Day 3
Meal 1	**Salmon and Kale Frittata** *p. 150* Calories 498 *Fat 40g | Carbs 7g | Protein 29g*	**Herb Scramble with Spicy Tomatoes and Mushrooms** *p. 145* Calories 369 *Fat 30g | Carbs 8g | Protein 18g*	**Mushroom Omelet** *p. 149* Calories 468 *Fat 39g | Carbs 6g | Protein 25g*
Meal 2	**Beef Cobb Salad with Chipotle Ranch Dressing** *p. 166* Calories 526 *Fat 37g | Carbs 12g | Protein 38g*	**Almond and Parmesan Chicken Salad** *p. 169* Calories 582 *Fat 47g | Carbs 14g | Protein 39g*	**Thai Beef Salad with Satay Dressing** *p. 170* Calories 446 *Fat 28g | Carbs 13g | Protein 37g*
Meal 3	**Red Chicken Curry with Zucchini Noodles** *p. 190* Calories 424 *Fat 32g | Carbs 15g | Protein 22g*	**One-Pan Mediterranean Pork** *p. 194* Calories 432 *Fat 31g | Carbs 9g | Protein 26g*	**Pork Lettuce Wraps with Spicy Cucumber Salad** *p. 174* Calories 533 *Fat 41g | Carbs 15g | Protein 27g*
Totals	**Calories 1,448 Fat 109g** (68%) **| Carbs 34g** (9%) *Fiber 7g* **| Protein 89g** (25%)	**Calories 1,383 Fat 108g** (70%) **| Carbs 31g** (9%) *Fiber 9g* **| Protein 83g** (24%)	**Calories 1,447 Fat 108g** (67%) **| Carbs 34g** (9%) *Fiber 9g* **| Protein 89g** (25%)

Parmesan Herb Crusted Salmon with Sautéed Spinach (page 188)

Day 4	Day 5	Day 6	Day 7
Vanilla Coconut "Oats" p. 138 Calories 356 *Fat 32g | Carbs 10g | Protein 10g*	**Avocado, Egg, and Salmon Toast** p. 142 Calories 499 *Fat 36g | Carbs 14g | Protein 30g*	**Herb Scramble with Spicy Tomatoes and Mushrooms** p. 145 Calories 369 *Fat 30g | Carbs 8g | Protein 18g*	**Mushroom Omelet** p. 149 Calories 468 *Fat 39g | Carbs 6g | Protein 25g*
Chicken Ranch Chop Salad p. 165 Calories 433 *Fat 27g | Carbs 12g | Protein 38g*	**Thai Beef Salad with Satay Dressing** p. 170 Calories 446 *Fat 28g | Carbs 13g | Protein 37g*	**Chicken and Goat Cheese Salad** p. 168 Calories 474 *Fat 35g | Carbs 11g | Protein 32g*	**Almond and Parmesan Chicken Salad** p. 169 Calories 582 *Fat 47g | Carbs 14g | Protein 39g*
Peppery Ginger Beef and Broccoli Stir-Fry p. 176 Calories 411 *Fat 24g | Carbs 13g | Protein 36g* **Keto Coffee** p. 209 Calories 196 *Fat 22g | Carbs 0g | Protein 1g*	**One-Pan Creamy Tuscan Beef** p. 196 Calories 528 *Fat 46g | Carbs 8g | Protein 25g*	**One-Pan Mediterranean Pork** p. 194 Calories 432 *Fat 31g | Carbs 9g | Protein 26g* **Keto Coffee** p. 209 Calories 196 *Fat 22g | Carbs 0g | Protein 1g*	**Parmesan Herb Crusted Salmon with Sautéed Spinach** p. 188 Calories 432 *Fat 23g | Carbs 15g | Protein 32g*
Calories 1,396 **Fat 105g** (68%) | **Carbs 35g** (10%) *Fiber 15g* | **Protein 85g** (24%)	**Calories 1,473** **Fat 110g** (67%) | **Carbs 35g** (10%) *Fiber 13g* | **Protein 92g** (25%)	**Calories 1,471** **Fat 118g** (72%) | **Carbs 28g** (8%) *Fiber 8g* | **Protein 77g** (21%)	**Calories 1,482** **Fat 109g** (66%) | **Carbs 35g** (9%) *Fiber 14g* | **Protein 96g** (26%)

DAIRY-FREE MEAL PLAN

Dairy foods don't agree with everyone. For those who don't feel their best when they eat dairy products, this 3-day meal plan shows you how to eat a low-carb diet without common high-fat dairy foods such as cheese and cream.

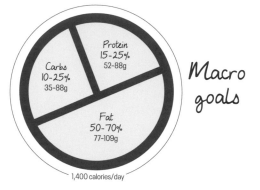

Protein
15-25%
52-88g

Carbs
10-25%
35-88g

Fat
50-70%
77-109g

Macro goals

1,400 calories/day

How to Do It

- Create a weekly shopping list, and prep food ahead of time. Have low-carb dairy-free snacks ready, such as hard-boiled eggs, avocados, nuts, or nonstarchy veggies.

- See page 121 for instructions specific to your fasting plan.

- You can add nondairy fats such as MCT or coconut oil to coffee or tea, but you'll want to account for the calories. Nut milks are a nondairy option, but they contain nutrients that could break your fast, so you'll want to account for the calories and consume these only during your eating window.

3-day schedule	**Day 1**	**Day 2**	**Day 3**
Meal 1	Chocolate Coconut "Oats" *p. 138* Calories 399 *Fat 33g	Carbs 19g	Protein 11g*	Sautéed Mushroom and Spinach Toast *p. 137* Calories 399 *Fat 30g	Carbs 16g	Protein 21g*	Smoked Salmon with Egg and Asparagus *p. 136* Calories 262 *Fat 19g	Carbs 12g	Protein 17g*
Meal 2	Grilled Green Goodness Salad *p. 158* Calories 477 *Fat 30g	Carbs 31g	Protein 27g*	Charred Broccoli and Salmon Salad with Tahini Dressing *p. 154* Calories 487 *Fat 36g	Carbs 36g	Protein 14g*	Turkey and Avocado Asian Cabbage Salad *p. 160* Calories 621 *Fat 46g	Carbs 29g	Protein 28g*
Meal 3	One-Pan Prosciutto-Wrapped Shrimp and Broccoli *p. 180* Calories 512 *Fat 36g	Carbs 23g	Protein 28g*	Spicy Chicken and Eggplant *p. 181* Calories 456 *Fat 30g	Carbs 22g	Protein 28g*	Pork, Pepper, and Cabbage Stir-Fry *p. 177* Calories 493 *Fat 28g	Carbs 22g	Protein 40g* - - - - - - - - - ½ cup blueberries *(per person; eat any time of day)* Calories 42 *Fat 0g	Carbs 9g	Protein 1g*
Totals	Calories 1,388 **Fat 99g** (64%) **| Carbs 73g** (21%) *Fiber 29g* **| Protein 66g** (19%)	Calories 1,342 **Fat 96g** (64%) **| Carbs 74g** (22%) *Fiber 25g* **| Protein 63g** (19%)	Calories 1,418 **Fat 93g** (59%) **| Carbs 72g** (20%) *Fiber 23g* **| Protein 86g** (24%)

VEGETARIAN MEAL PLAN

There are many different ways to follow a vegetarian diet; this plan omits meat and fish but includes eggs and dairy for protein. Getting adequate protein is a challenge for vegetarians, so you may find it necessary to supplement with plant-based protein powder.

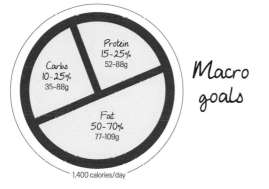

Protein
15-25%
52-88g

Carbs
10-25%
35-88g

Fat
50-70%
77-109g

Macro goals

1,400 calories/day

How to Do It

- Create a weekly shopping list, and prep food ahead of time. Have low-carb vegetarian snacks ready, such as hard-boiled eggs, avocados, nuts, cheese, full-fat plain yogurt, or nonstarchy veggies.

- See page 121 for instructions specific to your fasting plan.

- You will feel your best if you consume a low-carb protein powder drink during your eating window to reach your goal macros. Look for a product that offers about 20 grams of protein per serving.

- You can add cream and other fats to coffee, but you'll want to account for the calories.

3-day schedule	Day 1	Day 2	Day 3
Meal 1	**Herb Scramble with Spicy Tomatoes and Mushrooms** *p. 145* Calories 369 *Fat 30g | Carbs 8g | Protein 18g*	**Chocolate Coconut "Oats"** *p. 138* Calories 399 *Fat 33g | Carbs 19g | Protein 11g*	**Blueberry Lime Almond Muffins** *p. 141* *(2 muffins/person)* Calories 564 *Fat 50g | Carbs 22g | Protein 16g*
Meal 2	**Charred Broccoli Salad with Tahini Dressing** *(vegetarian variation)* *p. 154* Calories 501 *Fat 34g | Carbs 43g | Protein 17g*	**Spicy Chickpea Salad** *p. 156* Calories 645 *Fat 46g | Carbs 42g | Protein 22g*	**Grilled Green Goodness Salad** *(vegetarian variation)* *p. 159* Calories 477 *Fat 34g | Carbs 32g | Protein 18g*
Meal 3	**Mushroom and Swiss "Burgers"** *p. 185* Calories 506 *Fat 38g | Carbs 29g | Protein 19g*	**Quick and Easy Vegetable Curry** *p. 182* Calories 357 *Fat 22g | Carbs 28g | Protein 9g*	**Broccolini and Roasted Pepper Quiche** *p. 144* Calories 360 *Fat 23g | Carbs 20g | Protein 21g*
Totals	**Calories 1,376 Fat 102g** (67%) **| Carbs 80g** (23%) *Fiber 34g |* **Protein 54g** (16%)	**Calories 1,401 Fat 101g** (65%) **| Carbs 89g** (25%) *Fiber 28g |* **Protein 42g** (12%)	**Calories 1,401 Fat 107g** (69%) **| Carbs 74g** (21%) *Fiber 23g |* **Protein 55g** (16%)

8

EGGS + LOW-CARB TWISTS ON GRAINS

Everyone loves pancakes, and you can even eat them on a low-carb diet using almond flour and stevia. With three fluffy pancakes per serving, you will feel totally satisfied.

VANILLA CINNAMON PANCAKES

MAKES: 6 PANCAKES　　**PREP: 10 MINUTES**　　**COOK: 20 MINUTES**

⅔ cup blanched almond flour

1 tbsp stevia or granulated monk fruit sweetener

1 tsp baking powder

½ tsp ground cinnamon

2 large eggs

2oz (56g) cream cheese, softened

2 tsp pure vanilla extract

Sea salt, to taste

Butter, blueberries, and full-fat yogurt (optional), for serving

1 In the bowl of a food processor, add the almond flour, stevia, baking powder, cinnamon, eggs, cream cheese, vanilla, and salt. Process until smooth. Let stand for 5 minutes to thicken slightly.

2 Heat a lightly greased nonstick griddle pan to medium or a nonstick skillet over medium heat. Pour a scant 3 tablespoons batter for each pancake onto the griddle to make 6 pancakes. Cook for 2 minutes or until bubbles appear on the surface. Carefully flip the pancakes over. Cook for 1 minute or until browned.

3 Serve the pancakes immediately with butter, blueberries, and yogurt (if using).

Bypass the maple syrup by defrosting a cup of frozen blueberries in the microwave for about 90 seconds. As they warm, the juices form a syrup you can drizzle.

NUTRITION PER 3 PANCAKES (excluding options for serving)

CALORIES: **384**　　FAT: **34g**　　CARBOHYDRATES: **16g**　　FIBER: **3g**　　SUGARS: **3g**　　PROTEIN: **15g**

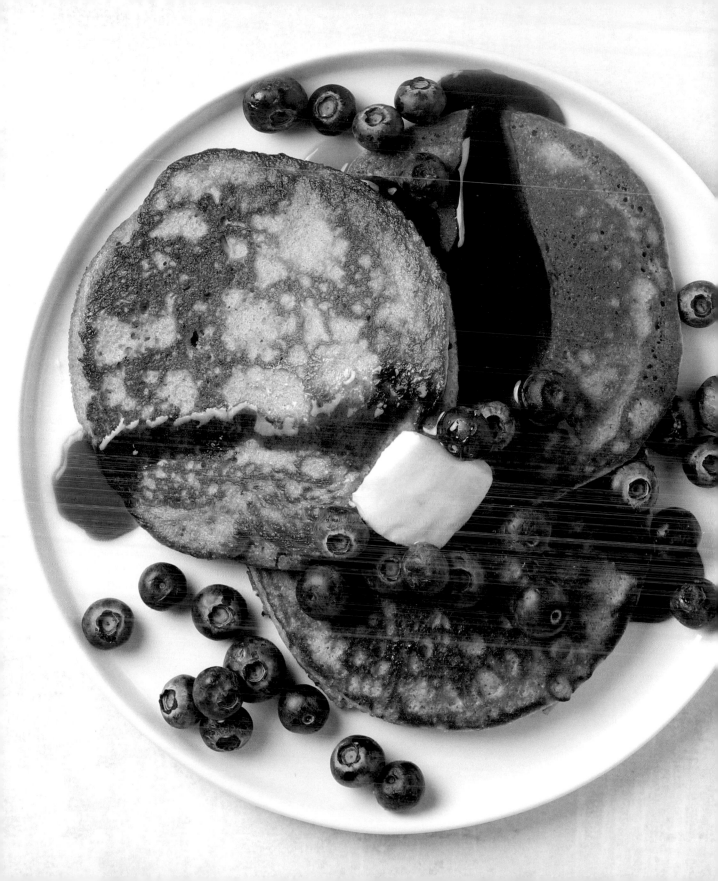

AMP UP THE FAT AND PROTEIN:
ADD MORE SMOKED SALMON OR EGGS.

GF

Simple ingredients—sweet tomatoes, vibrant asparagus, smoked salmon, and fried eggs with crispy, golden, lacy edges—come together to make a lovely breakfast or brunch.

SMOKED SALMON WITH EGG AND ASPARAGUS

SERVES: **2**   PREP: **5 MINUTES**   COOK: **15 MINUTES**

2 tbsp butter, divided

8oz (226g) cherry or grape tomatoes

Sea salt and freshly ground black pepper, to taste

1 tsp balsamic vinegar

2 large eggs

14 asparagus spears, trimmed of woody ends and halved crosswise

3oz (85g) thinly sliced smoked salmon

Chopped dill (optional), for garnish

Lemon wedges, for serving

1 In a medium skillet, melt 1 tablespoon butter over medium-high heat. Add the tomatoes, and season with salt and pepper. Cook, stirring occasionally, for 3 minutes. Using a potato masher, gently press down on the tomatoes to pop them. Add the vinegar. Cook for 2 to 3 minutes, stirring occasionally, until the juices are thickened. Cover to keep warm, and set aside.

2 While the tomatoes are cooking, in a separate small skillet, melt the remaining 1 tablespoon butter over medium heat until hot. Crack the eggs into the melted butter, and cook the eggs for 5 minutes, without turning, until the whites are set and the outside edges have become lacy and crispy.

3 Boil, steam, or microwave the asparagus for about 3 minutes or until tender-crisp. (To microwave, place in a small baking dish with about 1 tablespoon water, cover, and microwave on high for 3 minutes.)

4 To assemble, arrange the asparagus on two plates. Top with the tomato mixture, smoked salmon, and eggs. Sprinkle with pepper and dill (if using), and serve immediately alongside lemon wedges.

NUTRITION PER SERVING

CALORIES: **262**   FAT: **19g**   CARBOHYDRATES: **12g**   FIBER: **3g**   SUGARS: **5g**   PROTEIN: **17g**

You will love this low-carb toast piled high with sautéed mushrooms, baby spinach, and an egg cooked to perfection. Enjoy for a leisurely weekend brunch or a substantial breakfast midweek.

SAUTÉED MUSHROOM AND SPINACH TOAST

🍴 SERVES: **2**   🕐 PREP: **10 MINUTES**   🔥 COOK: **10 MINUTES**

1½ tbsp olive oil, divided

8oz (226g) small brown mushrooms, sliced

½ tsp garlic powder

Sea salt, to taste

½ tsp freshly ground black pepper

4oz (113g) baby spinach leaves (about 5 cups)

2 large eggs

2 slices of Low-Carb Bread Loaf (page 205)

2 tsp spicy brown mustard

1 In a large skillet, heat 1 tablespoon oil over medium-high heat. Add the mushrooms, garlic powder, salt, and pepper. Cook, stirring occasionally, for 5 minutes or until the mushrooms are browned. Remove to a bowl. Cover to keep warm.

2 In the same skillet, cook the spinach over medium-high heat, stirring, for 1 to 2 minutes or until the spinach is just wilted. Season to taste with salt and pepper.

3 Meanwhile, in a separate small nonstick skillet, heat the remaining ½ tablespoon oil over medium-high heat. Add the eggs, and cook to your liking—about 4 minutes for sunny side up.

4 While the eggs are cooking, toast the bread. Spread the mustard on the toast. Arrange the mushrooms and then the spinach on the slices of toast, and top each slice with an egg. Serve immediately.

NUTRITION PER SERVING

CALORIES: **399**   FAT: **30g**   CARBOHYDRATES: **16g**   FIBER: **4g**   SUGARS: **5g**   PROTEIN: **21g**

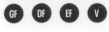

Chia and hempseeds make a delicious lower-carb alternative to oats. Enjoy the decadent chocolate version with oranges and berries, or make the vanilla variation for something even lower in carbs.

CHOCOLATE COCONUT "OATS"

SERVES: **2**　　　PREP: **5 MINUTES**　　　COOK: **NONE**

¼ cup unsweetened coconut flakes

3 tbsp chia seeds

3 tbsp plus 1 tsp hempseeds, divided

1 tbsp cacao powder

1 tbsp stevia or granulated monk fruit sweetener

Sea salt, to taste

1 cup (250ml) full-fat coconut milk (such as A Taste of Thai), chilled

2 tbsp ice water

1 cup sliced strawberries (hulled)

1 mandarin orange, segmented

1 tbsp cacao nibs

Coconut flakes and assorted berries (optional), for serving

1 In a small bowl, combine the coconut, chia seeds, 3 tablespoons hempseeds, cacao powder, stevia, and salt.

2 Add the chilled coconut milk, ice water, strawberry slices, and mandarin segments. Stir to combine. Let stand for 5 minutes before serving.

3 Divide the "oats" into serving bowls. Sprinkle with the remaining 1 teaspoon hempseeds and the cacao nibs. Top with extra coconut and berries (if using).

For Vanilla Coconut "Oats": In step 1, stir in ½ teaspoon pure vanilla extract and omit the cacao powder.
In step 2, omit the 1 cup sliced strawberries and the mandarin orange.

This recipe will keep for 4 days in a sealed container in the refrigerator; add extra coconut milk or water if the oats have thickened too much.

NUTRITION PER SERVING FOR CHOCOLATE COCONUT "OATS"
(excluding options for serving)

CALORIES: **399**　FAT: **33g**　CARBOHYDRATES: **19g**　FIBER: **8g**　SUGARS: **6g**　PROTEIN: **11g**

NUTRITION PER SERVING FOR VANILLA COCONUT "OATS"
(excluding options for serving)

CALORIES: **356**　FAT: **32g**　CARBOHYDRATES: **10g**　FIBER: **7g**　SUGARS: **3g**　PROTEIN: **10g**

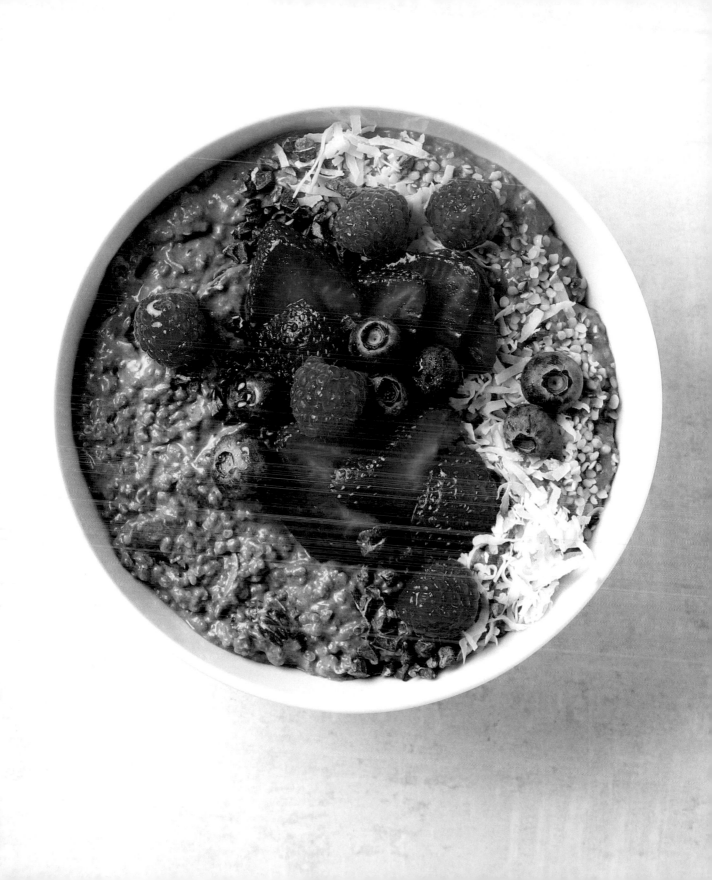

Cacao powder gives these muffins a deep chocolate flavor that goes perfectly with the fresh raspberries and pecans. Eat the muffins fresh from the oven, or freeze them so you'll always have a quick snack on hand.

GRAB-AND-GO CHOCOLATE BERRY MUFFINS

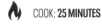

MAKES: 12 MUFFINS   **PREP: 10 MINUTES**   **COOK: 25 MINUTES**

1¾ cups blanched almond flour

⅓ cup stevia or granulated monk fruit sweetener

¼ cup whole psyllium husks

¼ cup cacao or cocoa powder

2 tsp baking powder

Sea salt, to taste

1 cup raspberries (or other fresh berries, such as blueberries or chopped strawberries)

½ cup chopped pecans

3 large eggs

⅓ cup plain whole milk yogurt or coconut yogurt

⅓ cup avocado oil or melted coconut oil

1 Preheat the oven to 400°F (200°C). Line a 12-cup muffin pan with liners.

2 In a large bowl, combine the almond flour, stevia, psyllium, cacao powder, baking powder, and salt. Add the raspberries and pecans. Mix to combine.

3 In a medium bowl, whisk together the eggs, yogurt, and oil. Add the egg mixture to the flour mixture and stir until the mixture just comes together.

4 Spoon the mixture into the muffin cups at least three-fourths full. (An ice cream scoop works well for this.) Bake for 20 to 25 minutes or until a toothpick inserted into the center of a muffin comes out clean. Let stand in the pan for 5 minutes before removing the muffins to a wire rack to cool. Serve warm or at room temperature.

To store, wrap the cooled muffins tightly in plastic wrap. Freeze for up to 3 months. Leave to thaw at room temperature, or microwave for 20 seconds.

NUTRITION PER MUFFIN

CALORIES: **257**   FAT: **22g**   CARBOHYDRATES: **12g**   FIBER: **7g**   SUGARS: **2g**   PROTEIN: **6g**

These subtly sweet muffins are easy to make. The juicy, sweet blueberries pop in your mouth with a hint of tart lime. Substitute the lime zest with lemon zest, if preferred.

BLUEBERRY LIME ALMOND MUFFINS

MAKES: 12 MUFFINS   **PREP: 10 MINUTES**   **COOK: 25 MINUTES**

3 cups blanched almond flour

¼ cup coconut flour

2 tbsp baking powder

½ tsp xanthan gum

½ tsp baking soda

⅓ cup stevia or granulated monk fruit sweetener

Sea salt, to taste

1 cup blueberries

1 cup whole milk or almond milk

½ cup avocado oil or melted butter

2 large eggs

2 tbsp finely grated lime zest

1 tsp pure vanilla extract

Sliced almonds (optional), for topping

1 Preheat the oven to 375°F (190°C). Line a 12-cup muffin pan with liners.

2 In a large bowl, whisk together the almond flour, coconut flour, baking powder, xanthan gum, baking soda, stevia, and salt until combined.

3 Add the blueberries, and stir to combine with the flour mixture.

4 In a medium bowl, whisk together the milk, oil, eggs, zest, and vanilla. Add the milk mixture to the flour mixture. Stir until the ingredients are just combined.

5 Spoon the mixture into the muffin cups at least three-fourths full. (An ice cream scoop works well for this.) Sprinkle with the sliced almonds (if using). Bake for 25 minutes or until the muffins are browned and a toothpick inserted into the center of a muffin comes out clean. Let stand in the pan for 5 minutes before removing the muffins to a wire rack to cool. Serve warm or at room temperature.

To store, wrap the cooled muffins tightly in plastic wrap. Freeze for up to 3 months. Leave to thaw at room temperature, or microwave for 45 seconds.

NUTRITION PER MUFFIN

CALORIES: **282**   FAT: **25g**   CARBOHYDRATES: **11g**   FIBER: **4g**   SUGARS: **3g**   PROTEIN: **8g**

There are few better breakfast combinations than avocado, smoked salmon, and eggs. The mashed avocado is flavored with lemon and chives and slathered over low-carb toast. The smoked salmon is piled on, then topped with poached eggs and drizzled with your favorite hot sauce.

AVOCADO, EGG, AND SALMON TOAST

SERVES: **2**   PREP: **10 MINUTES**   COOK: **5 MINUTES**

½ avocado, sliced

1 tbsp fresh lemon juice

2 tsp snipped chives, plus extra for garnish

Sea salt and freshly ground black pepper, to taste

2 tbsp white vinegar

4 large eggs

2 slices of Low-Carb Bread Loaf (page 205)

1 cup baby spinach leaves

3oz (85g) smoked salmon

⅓ cup crumbled feta cheese

1 tsp hot sauce (optional), for serving

1 In a small bowl, mash the avocado with a fork. Add the lemon juice, chives, salt, and pepper. Mix until well combined.

2 In a small sauté pan, bring 3 inches (7.5cm) water to a boil. Reduce to a simmer. Add the vinegar. Dropping in one egg at a time, crack the egg into a small ramekin or cup, and carefully pour into the simmering water from just above the water level. Poach the eggs (all at once) for 4 minutes for soft yolks. Using a slotted spoon, carefully remove the eggs from the water to a small paper towel–lined plate to drain.

3 While the eggs are cooking, toast the bread. Cut each slice of toast in half, and spread with the avocado mixture. Place two halves on two serving plates. Top with spinach, salmon, and the eggs. Season with salt and pepper. Scatter the feta over the eggs, and drizzle with the hot sauce (if using). Garnish with extra chives, and serve immediately.

NUTRITION PER SERVING

CALORIES: **499**   FAT: **36g**   CARBOHYDRATES: **14g**   FIBER: **8g**   SUGARS: **3g**   PROTEIN: **30g**

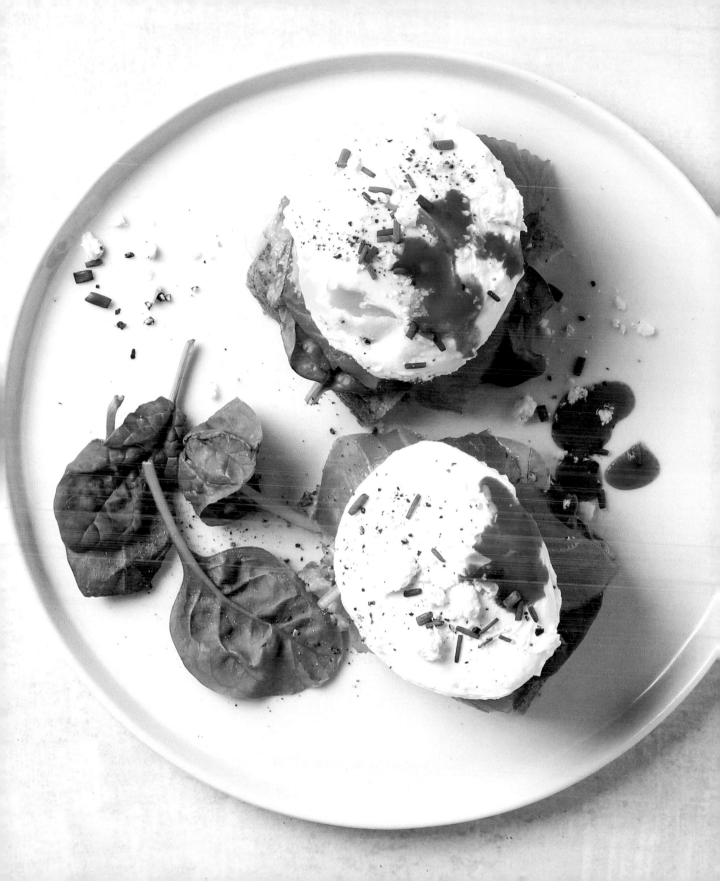

This is a rich and creamy quiche with a tasty medley of broccolini, spinach, and red pepper. It can be made a day ahead, covered, and refrigerated.

BROCCOLINI AND ROASTED PEPPER QUICHE

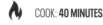

⚔ SERVES: **3**   🕐 PREP: **12 MINUTES**   🔥 COOK: **40 MINUTES**

1 bunch Broccolini (about 6 pieces), or 8oz (226g) sliced broccoli

1 tbsp butter

2 garlic cloves, minced

1 cup baby spinach leaves

1 roasted red pepper, chopped (about ½ cup)

1 cup cooked great northern beans

4oz (113g) crumbled feta cheese, divided

8 large eggs

⅔ cup sour cream or crème fraiche

¼ tsp ground nutmeg

Sea salt and freshly ground black pepper, to taste

¼ cup chopped basil leaves, plus extra for garnish

1 Grease a deep 9-inch (23cm) pie dish. Preheat the oven to 350°F (180°C).

2 Place the Broccolini in a microwave-safe container. Add about 2 tablespoons water, cover with plastic wrap, and microwave on full power for 2 to 3 minutes or until the Broccolini is bright green and tender-crisp; do not boil or overcook. Place on a paper towel to absorb excess moisture.

3 In a small skillet, melt the butter over medium-low heat. Add the garlic, and cook, stirring, for 1 minute until softened and fragrant.

4 Add the spinach. Cook, stirring, for 1 to 2 minutes or until the leaves are just wilted. Spoon the spinach mixture into the pie dish. Arrange the Broccolini, roasted red peppers, and beans in the same dish. Sprinkle with half of the feta.

5 In a medium bowl, whisk together the eggs, sour cream, nutmeg, salt, and pepper until well combined.

6 Slowly pour the egg mixture into the dish over the vegetables. Sprinkle with the remaining feta and the basil. Bake in the middle part of the oven for 35 minutes or until the top is a little puffed and the quiche is set when gently jiggled. Let cool for 1 to 2 hours. (The quiche will set further when cooled.) Serve warm or cold. (It is easier to cut once when cool.) Cut into three wedges. Garnish with extra basil leaves.

NUTRITION PER SERVING

CALORIES: **360**   FAT: **23g**   CARBOHYDRATES: **20g**   FIBER: **5g**   SUGARS: **4g**   PROTEIN: **21g**

These creamy cheese and herb scrambled eggs are served with sautéed tomatoes and mushrooms with a hint of chili. This scramble would make a perfect weekend brunch.

HERB SCRAMBLE WITH SPICY TOMATOES AND MUSHROOMS

SERVES: **2**   PREP: **5 MINUTES**   COOK: **8 MINUTES**

1 tbsp butter

4 large eggs

2 tbsp heavy cream

1 tbsp chopped dill, plus extra sprigs for garnish

1 tbsp chopped flat-leaf parsley

Sea salt, to taste

¼ cup grated white Cheddar cheese

Microgreens (optional), for serving

Spicy tomatoes and mushrooms:

1 tbsp butter

6oz (170g) grape or cherry tomatoes

6oz (170g) brown mushrooms, quartered

Pinch of crushed red pepper

Sea salt and freshly ground black pepper, to taste

1 Make the spicy tomatoes and mushrooms. In a medium or large skillet, melt the butter over medium-high heat. Add the tomatoes and mushrooms. Cook, stirring occasionally, until the tomatoes are blistered and the mushrooms are browned, about 5 minutes.

2 Add the crushed red pepper, salt, and pepper. Cook, stirring, until combined.

3 While the tomatoes and mushrooms are cooking, prepare the eggs. In a small nonstick skillet, melt the butter over medium-low heat.

4 In a medium bowl, whisk together the eggs, cream, dill, parsley, and salt. Pour into the skillet. Sprinkle the Cheddar over the eggs. Cook, stirring occasionally, for 3 minutes or until almost set. Turn off the heat and fold the egg gently until just cooked.

5 Serve the eggs immediately with the tomato mixture, extra dill sprigs, and microgreens (if using).

NUTRITION PER SERVING

CALORIES: **369**   FAT: **30g**   CARBOHYDRATES: **8g**   FIBER: **1g**   SUGARS: **4g**   PROTEIN: **18g**

Crispy kale, runny yolks, and plenty of creamy avocado tastes amazing with the spicy harissa. Serve this for breakfast or brunch or as a perfect light and easy dinner. It's delicious sprinkled with your favorite cheese—feta, Parmesan, Cheddar, or a smoked variety.

TOMATO BAKED EGGS

SERVES: 2   **PREP: 15 MINUTES**   **COOK: 25 MINUTES**

1½ tbsp avocado oil

½ cup diced red onion

½ cup diced red bell pepper

2 garlic cloves, minced

2 tbsp tomato paste

2 tsp harissa paste (a North African chili paste, or use a pinch of crushed red pepper)

1 tsp smoked paprika

¼ tsp ground cumin

1 (14oz/396g) can fire-roasted diced tomatoes, undrained

Sea salt and freshly ground black pepper, to taste

4 large eggs

1 cup torn kale leaves

⅓ cup crumbled feta cheese, or another favorite cheese such as Parmesan, Cheddar, or smoked Gouda

1 avocado, sliced

2 tbsp coarsely chopped cilantro

1 Preheat the oven to 375°F (190°C). In a large oven-safe skillet, such as a 10-inch (25cm) cast-iron skillet, heat the oil over medium heat. Add the onion, bell pepper, and garlic. Cook, stirring occasionally, for 5 minutes or until the onion and pepper are softened.

2 Add the tomato paste, harissa, paprika, and cumin. Cook, stirring, for 30 seconds, or until fragrant.

3 Add the tomatoes with their juices, salt, and pepper. Cook, uncovered, stirring occasionally, for 5 to 7 minutes or until the sauce thickens. Remove from the heat.

4 Make four indents evenly spaced in the sauce, and crack an egg into each indent. Place the kale around the eggs and the edge of skillet. Sprinkle with salt and pepper.

5 Bake for 12 minutes or until the egg whites are cooked but the yolks are still soft. Top with feta, avocado, and cilantro, and serve immediately straight from the pan.

NUTRITION PER SERVING

CALORIES: **330**   FAT: **20g**   CARBOHYDRATES: **23g**   FIBER: **5g**   SUGARS: **11g**   PROTEIN: **16g**

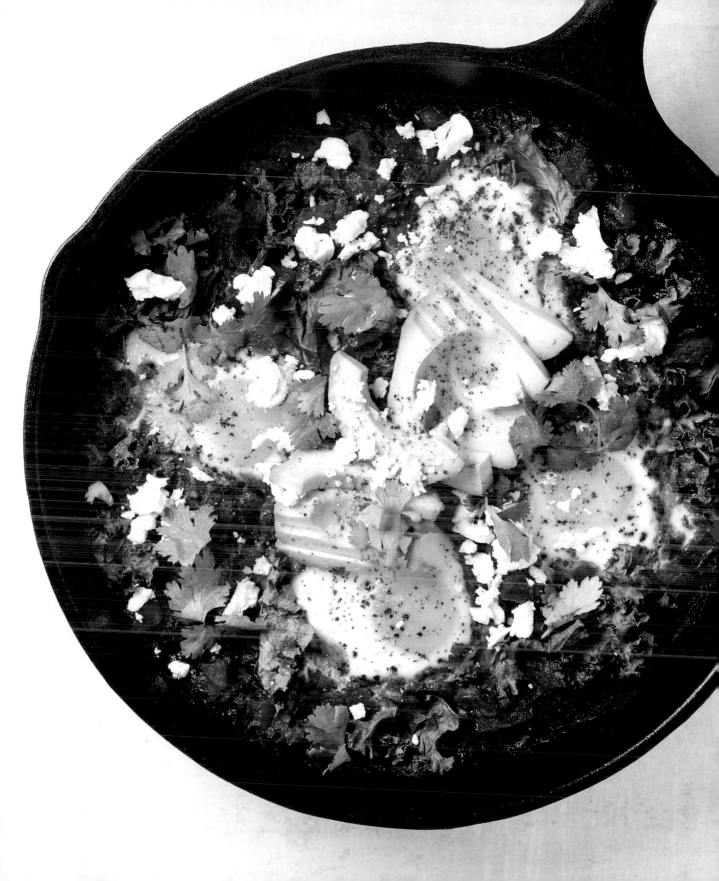

This rich omelet has plenty of cheese and meat and is topped with pico de gallo and cilantro to complete the flavor profile. Make one larger omelet and cut in half to serve, or cook in two very small skillets, if you have them.

MEXICAN OMELET

✕ SERVES: **2**   🕐 PREP: **20 MINUTES**   🔥 COOK: **20 MINUTES**

1 tsp avocado oil

¼lb (113g) ground beef

1 tsp fajita seasoning

¼ cup plus 1 tbsp water, divided

3 large eggs

Sea salt and freshly ground black pepper, to taste

1 tsp butter

⅓ cup grated pepper jack cheese

2 tbsp sour cream (optional)

½ avocado, sliced

2 tbsp sliced pickled jalapeños (such as Mezzetta), drained

½ cup pico de gallo (page 184 or store-bought), or sliced tomatoes

Cilantro sprigs, for garnish

1 In a medium skillet, heat the oil over medium-high heat. Add the beef and cook, stirring and breaking up any lumps, for 5 to 8 minutes or until browned. Add the fajita seasoning and stir to combine. Add ¼ cup water and continue to cook, stirring occasionally, until most of the liquid has evaporated. Set aside.

2 In a medium bowl, whisk together the eggs, salt, pepper, and the remaining 1 tablespoon water. In a separate 8-inch (20cm) nonstick skillet, melt the butter over medium heat. Add the egg mixture and reduce the heat to medium-low. Cook, covered, for 3 to 5 minutes or until the eggs are just set and the omelet is golden brown on the bottom.

3 Sprinkle one half of the omelet with the pepper jack. Spoon the beef mixture over the cheese. Fold the other side of the omelet over to cover the filling. Slide the omelet from the pan to a warm board or plate, and cut in half. Place the halves on two serving plates.

4 Top with equal amounts sour cream (if using), avocado, jalapeño slices, pico de gallo, and cilantro sprigs. Serve immediately.

NUTRITION PER SERVING

CALORIES: **450**   FAT: **35g**   CARBOHYDRATES: **13g**   FIBER: **4g**   SUGARS: **7g**   PROTEIN: **24g**

You can really add almost any ingredients to an omelet. This one uses sautéed mushrooms, chives, fresh mozzarella, and Gruyère cheese, but mix it up if you'd like to! Serve the omelet open or folded.

MUSHROOM OMELET

SERVES: **1**   PREP: **10 MINUTES**   COOK: **10 MINUTES**

1 tbsp avocado oil

4oz (113g) small brown mushrooms, sliced

2 large eggs

2 tbsp snipped chives, plus extra for garnish

Sea salt and freshly ground black pepper, to taste

Pinch of ground nutmeg

1oz (28g) fresh mozzarella cheese, torn

¼ cup shredded Gruyère cheese, divided

1 In an 8-inch (20cm) nonstick skillet, heat the oil over medium-high heat. Add the mushrooms. Cook, stirring occasionally, for 3 to 4 minutes or until softened.

2 In a small bowl, whisk together eggs, chives, salt, pepper, and nutmeg until combined. Pour into the skillet. Add the mozzarella and half of the Gruyère. Reduce the heat to medium and cook for 3 minutes, swirling the pan and lifting the edge of the omelet to allow the egg to flow underneath. Continue until the uncooked egg from the top is mostly gone.

3 Sprinkle with the remaining Gruyère. Cook for 1 to 2 minutes more or until the omelet is set. Sprinkle with extra chives. Serve the omelet open or folded.

NUTRITION PER SERVING

CALORIES: **468**   FAT: **39g**   CARBOHYDRATES: **6g**   FIBER: **1g**   SUGARS: **3g**   PROTEIN: **25g**

AMP UP THE FAT AND PROTEIN:

SERVE WITH SLICED AVOCADO OR EXTRA RICOTTA.

GF

This frittata is perfect for a hearty breakfast, a delicious lunch, or a light dinner. The ricotta and fresh dill make it light and summery.

SALMON AND KALE FRITTATA

SERVES: 3   **PREP: 10 MINUTES**   **COOK: 25 MINUTES**

6 large eggs

½ cup heavy whipping cream

2 tbsp chopped dill, plus extra for garnish

Pinch of ground nutmeg

Sea salt and freshly ground black pepper, to taste

1 tbsp avocado oil

2 cups (2oz/60g) shredded kale leaves

4oz (113g) cooked skin-off salmon, flaked

½ cup ricotta cheese

⅓ cup grated white Cheddar cheese

1 Preheat the oven to 400°F (200°C). In a medium bowl, whisk together the eggs, cream, dill, nutmeg, salt, and pepper.

2 Heat an 8-inch (20cm) nonstick oven-safe skillet over medium heat. Add the oil and swirl to coat the base and edges of the skillet.

3 Add the kale and cook for 2 to 3 minutes or until just wilted.

4 Add the salmon to the skillet. Pour in the egg mixture, swirling the pan to ensure the mixture is evenly distributed. Spoon the ricotta over the top of the mixture. Sprinkle with the Cheddar. Reduce the heat to low. Cook, uncovered, for 7 minutes or until the edges start to set.

5 Place the skillet in the oven, uncovered, and bake for 15 minutes or until the frittata is set. Let cool in the pan. (You can slide the frittata onto a plate or serve it in the pan.)

6 Sprinkle with extra dill. Cut into three wedges and serve.

NUTRITION PER SERVING

CALORIES: **498**   FAT: **40g**   CARBOHYDRATES: **7g**   FIBER: **1g**   SUGARS: **1g**   PROTEIN: **29g**

This frittata makes a good make-ahead meal served cold or warmed in the microwave. The veggies, plenty of creamy cheese, and a burst of flavor from the basil are totally satisfying.

MUSHROOM AND ASPARAGUS FRITTATA

SERVES: 2   **PREP: 15 MINUTES**   **COOK: 40 MINUTES**

4oz (113g) asparagus, trimmed of woody ends and halved crosswise

1 tsp butter, plus extra for greasing

8oz (226g) small brown mushrooms, sliced

4 large eggs

2 tbsp whole milk or cream

Sea salt and freshly ground black pepper, to taste

½ cup (0.5oz/14g) finely grated fresh Parmesan cheese

2 tbsp chopped basil, plus extra leaves for serving

⅓ cup ricotta cheese

1 cup cherry tomatoes, halved, for serving

1 Preheat the oven to 350°F (180°C). Bring a medium pan of water to a boil and reduce to a simmer. Plunge the asparagus into the pan of simmering water. Cook for 1 minute, or until bright green. Remove to a paper towel–lined plate.

2 In a small oven-safe nonstick frying pan (6–8in/15–20cm), melt the butter over medium-high heat. Cook the mushrooms in two batches until softened, about 5 minutes. Remove from the pan. Wipe the pan clean, and grease the bottom and sides with a little extra butter.

3 In a medium bowl, whisk together the eggs, milk, salt, and pepper. Add the Parmesan, basil, and mushrooms. Stir to combine.

4 Carefully pour the mixture into the pan. Arrange the asparagus in the egg mixture and dollop the ricotta over the top. Place the pan in the oven, uncovered, and bake for 30 minutes or until the frittata is set. Let cool in the pan. (You can slide the frittata onto a plate or serve it in the pan.)

5 Top with extra basil leaves. Cut into two wedges. Serve warm or cold with tomatoes on the side.

NUTRITION PER SERVING

CALORIES: **381**   FAT: **25g**   CARBOHYDRATES: **13g**   FIBER: **3g**   SUGARS: **5g**   PROTEIN: **32g**

9

BIG FAT SALADS

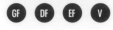
Creamy, veg-heavy, and delicious! Cook the salmon and vegetables on an outside grill for some extra smokiness, or indoors on a grill pan. This salad can be made vegetarian by adding canned cannellini beans and omitting the salmon.

CHARRED BROCCOLI AND SALMON SALAD WITH TAHINI DRESSING

SERVES: **1**   PREP: **15 MINUTES**   COOK: **12 MINUTES**

2oz (62g) skin-on salmon fillet

1½ tsp olive oil, divided

Sea salt and freshly ground black pepper, to taste

1 small red bell pepper, quartered, seeds and membranes removed

6oz (170g) broccoli, cut into slices or florets

4oz (110g) eggplant, sliced

3 cups baby spinach leaves

1 tbsp chopped walnuts, toasted

Lemon wedges (optional), for serving

Tahini dressing:

3 tbsp fresh lemon juice

1 tbsp olive oil

1 tbsp tahini

¼ tsp ground cumin

1 garlic clove, minced

Sea salt and freshly ground black pepper, to taste

1 Make the tahini dressing. In a small bowl, whisk together all of the ingredients until smooth.

2 Heat a grill or a grill pan to medium-high heat. Rub the salmon with ½ teaspoon oil and sprinkle with salt and pepper. Grill, skin-side down, for 4 minutes. Turn and cook for 3 minutes or until the salmon flakes easily with a fork. (Cooking time will vary depending on the thickness of the fillet.) Turn off the heat. Carefully remove the salmon to a plate. Remove and discard the skin; flake the salmon with a fork. Cover and set aside.

3 Heat the same grill or grill pan to medium-high heat. Cut the bell pepper sections into strips. In a medium bowl, toss together the remaining 1 teaspoon oil, pepper strips, broccoli, eggplant, and salt and pepper to taste. Cook for 3 minutes on each side until softened and grill marks appear. Halve the eggplant slices. Let the vegetables cool.

4 Place the spinach in a shallow serving bowl. Arrange the vegetables, flaked salmon, and walnuts over the spinach. Drizzle with the dressing and serve immediately with lemon wedges (if using).

Make it vegetarian: Swap the salmon with ¼ cup cooked cannellini beans (rinsed and drained if canned) or whatever legumes you prefer— lentils or navy beans make a good substitution. (This variation uses ½ teaspoon less olive oil.) Skip step 2. In step 4, arrange the beans along with the grilled vegetables and walnuts.

NUTRITION PER SERVING

CALORIES: **487**   FAT: **36g**   CARBOHYDRATES: **36g**   FIBER: **14g**   SUGARS: **14g**   PROTEIN: **14g**

NUTRITION PER SERVING (vegetarian variation)

CALORIES: **501**   FAT: **34g**   CARBOHYDRATES: **43g**   FIBER: **16g**   SUGARS: **14g**   PROTEIN: **17g**

You can make
the dressing and
the salad components
a day ahead of time
and assemble everything
just before serving.

AMP UP THE FAT AND PROTEIN: **ADD EXTRA FETA OR WALNUTS.**

GF **EF** **V**

Enjoy this vibrant salad with a lemony dressing and homemade crispy chickpeas. The salad packs easily for lunch on the go; just keep the chickpeas and the dressing separate until ready to eat.

SPICY CHICKPEA SALAD

SERVES: 1   **PREP: 15 MINUTES**   **COOK: 5 MINUTES**

1 tsp avocado oil or olive oil

1 (15oz/420g) can chickpeas, rinsed and drained

¼ tsp ground cumin

¼ tsp crushed red pepper

Sea salt and freshly ground black pepper, to taste

1 small head purple lettuce, trimmed and leaves separated

8 grape or cherry tomatoes, halved

1 small cucumber, sliced

½ roasted red pepper, sliced

¼ cup chopped flat-leaf parsley

6 thinly sliced red onion wedges

5 large green olives

2oz (60g) feta cheese, thinly sliced or crumbled

¼ cup (25g) raw walnuts

Lemon dressing:

2 tsp olive oil

1½ tbsp fresh lemon juice

¼ tsp ground cumin

1 small garlic clove, minced

Pinch of stevia or granulated monk fruit sweetener (optional)

Sea salt and freshly ground black pepper, to taste

1 Make the lemon dressing. In a jar with a screw-top lid, add all of the dressing ingredients. Shake until combined. Give the dressing another shake just before drizzling over the salad.

2 In a medium skillet, heat the oil over medium heat. Add the chickpeas, cumin, crushed red pepper, salt, and pepper. Cook, stirring occasionally, for 5 minutes or until the chickpeas are a little toasted and coated in the spice mixture. Let cool.

3 On a serving plate or shallow bowl, arrange the lettuce, tomatoes, cucumber, roasted red pepper slices, parsley, onion, and olives.

4 Scatter ½ cup chickpeas over the salad, reserving the remaining chickpeas for another use.

5 Drizzle with the dressing and top with the feta and walnuts. Serve immediately.

Store the leftover chickpeas in an airtight container in the refrigerator for up to 1 week. Enjoy as a snack or in salads, soups, and curries.

NUTRITION PER SERVING

CALORIES: **645**   FAT: **46g**   CARBOHYDRATES: **42g**   FIBER: **12g**   SUGARS: **15g**   PROTEIN: **22g**

Enjoy this delicious, colorful salad with a creamy horseradish, lemon, and caper dressing. Optionally, use cooked and flaked salmon in place of smoked salmon. You could serve with half of a low-carb Sesame Seed Bun (page 206) on the side to top it off!

SMOKED SALMON SALAD

✖️ SERVES: **1**   🕐 PREP: **15 MINUTES**   🔥 COOK: **NONE**

4 cups spring mix

5 radishes, thinly sliced

16 sugar snap peas, cut lengthwise into thirds or halves

2oz (57g) smoked salmon, cut into strips

¾ cup diced cucumber

4 tbsp diced red onion

Creamy horseradish dressing:

2 tbsp mayonnaise

2 tbsp fresh lemon juice

1 tsp prepared horseradish

1 tsp coarsely chopped, drained capers (heaping)

1 Make the creamy horseradish dressing. In a small bowl, whisk together all of the ingredients until combined.

2 On a serving plate or bowl, arrange the spring mix, radishes, sugar snap peas, salmon, cucumber, and onion. Spoon the dressing over the top and serve immediately.

NUTRITION PER SERVING

CALORIES: **348**   FAT: **23g**   CARBOHYDRATES: **16g**   FIBER: **3g**   SUGARS: **6g**   PROTEIN: **15g**

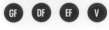
Baby spinach leaves topped with grilled vegetables and succulent salmon and drizzled with a cilantro-lime dressing makes a wholesome lunch or a light dinner. For a vegetarian version, serve with hard-boiled eggs instead of salmon.

GRILLED GREEN GOODNESS SALAD

SERVES: 2   **PREP: 20 MINUTES**   **COOK: 13 MINUTES**

6oz (170g) skin-on salmon fillet

2 tsp avocado oil, divided

Sea salt and freshly ground black pepper, to taste

5oz (142g) broccoli florets (about 2 cups)

5oz (141g) sugar snap peas, trimmed

10 asparagus spears, trimmed of woody ends

4 cups baby spinach leaves

1½ cups sliced strawberries (hulled)

4 scallions, thinly sliced

2 tbsp raw sunflower seeds

Cilantro-lime dressing:

3 tbsp fresh lime juice

3 tbsp chopped cilantro

2 tbsp avocado oil

1 tsp Dijon mustard

1 tsp coconut aminos

1 garlic clove

Pinch of stevia or granulated monk fruit sweetener (optional)

1 Make the cilantro-lime dressing. Place all of the ingredients in a small blender or food processor. Blend until smooth. Refrigerate until ready to use.

2 Preheat a grill or a grill pan to medium-high. Cut the salmon into two pieces. Brush ½ teaspoon oil over each fillet. Season with salt and pepper. Cook the salmon, skin-side down, for 3 minutes. Turn and cook for an additional 2 minutes or more or until the salmon flakes easily with a fork. (Cooking time will vary depending on the thickness of the fillets.) Turn off the heat. Remove the skin from the salmon, flake, and set aside.

3 Cut the broccoli lengthwise into ½-inch (1.25cm) thick slices. Preheat the same grill or grill pan to medium-high.

4 In a large bowl, toss together the broccoli, sugar snap peas, asparagus, remaining 1 teaspoon oil, and salt and pepper to taste until the vegetables are coated in oil. Cook in batches on the grill for 2 to 4 minutes per side or until grill marks appear and the vegetables are tender-crisp. Let cool. Cut the broccoli into smaller pieces, if desired.

5 Divide the spinach between two serving bowls, arrange the grilled vegetables over the top, add the flaked salmon, and drizzle with the dressing. Add the strawberries. Sprinkle with the scallions and sunflower seeds. Serve immediately.

NUTRITION PER SERVING

CALORIES: **477**   FAT: **30g**   CARBOHYDRATES: **31g**   FIBER: **10g**   SUGARS: **12g**   PROTEIN: **27g**

NUTRITION PER SERVING (vegetarian variation)

CALORIES: **477**   FAT: **34g**   CARBOHYDRATES: **32g**   FIBER: **10g**   SUGARS: **12g**   PROTEIN: **18g**

Make it vegetarian: Swap the salmon with 4 hard-boiled eggs (peeled; 2 per person). (This variation uses 1 teaspoon less avocado oil.) Skip step 2 and proceed with the remaining steps as written, adding the eggs in step 5.

GF DF EF

This salad is piled high with crunchy cabbage, celery, scallions, and almonds; topped with succulent turkey; and drizzled with a spicy ginger dressing.

TURKEY AND AVOCADO ASIAN CABBAGE SALAD

SERVES: 1   **PREP: 20 MINUTES**   **COOK: NONE**

2 cups finely shredded napa cabbage

1 cup finely shredded red cabbage

1 cup thinly sliced celery

¼ cup thinly sliced scallions

2 tbsp sliced almonds, toasted

2 tbsp coarsely chopped cilantro, plus extra for garnish

3oz (85g) cooked turkey or chicken breast, chopped

½ avocado, chopped

1 tsp sesame seeds, toasted

Spicy ginger dressing:

2 tbsp avocado oil

2 tbsp white wine vinegar

2 tsp grated ginger

1 tbsp coconut aminos

1 garlic clove

1 Make the spicy ginger dressing. In a small food processor or blender, process all of the ingredients until smooth.

2 In a medium bowl, toss together the napa cabbage, red cabbage, celery, scallions, almonds, cilantro, and turkey. Add half of the dressing, and toss to combine.

3 Pile the salad onto a serving plate. Top with the chopped avocado. Drizzle with the remaining dressing. Sprinkle with sesame seeds and extra cilantro for garnish. Serve immediately.

NUTRITION PER SERVING

CALORIES: **621**   FAT: **46g**   CARBOHYDRATES: **29g**   FIBER: **11g**   SUGARS: **9g**   PROTEIN: **28g**

This salad is loaded with a combination of fresh and crisp ingredients: tomatoes, cucumbers, and herbs drizzled in an olive dressing. It can easily be doubled to feed more people. Use the meatball recipe from page 192.

MEATBALL HERB SALAD WITH OLIVE DRESSING

SERVES: **1**   PREP: **15 MINUTES**   COOK: **NONE**

4 cups spring mix

6oz (170g) cherry or grape tomatoes, halved

¾ cup English cucumber slices

6 thin slices red onion

6 cooked meatballs, sliced, warmed if desired (such as the Greek Meatballs on page 192)

2 tbsp crumbled feta cheese

2 tbsp coarsely chopped walnuts, toasted

2 tbsp coarsely chopped mint leaves

2 tbsp coarsely chopped flat-leaf parsley

Olive dressing:

2 tbsp finely chopped pitted Kalamata olives

1 tbsp olive oil

1 tbsp balsamic vinegar

1 tbsp fresh lemon juice

1 garlic clove, minced

¼ tsp freshly ground black pepper

1 Make the olive dressing. In a small bowl, whisk together all of the ingredients.

2 On a serving plate, arrange the spring mix, tomatoes, cucumber, onion, and meatballs. Drizzle with the dressing. Sprinkle with the feta, walnuts, mint, and parsley. Toss to combine and serve immediately.

NUTRITION PER SERVING

CALORIES: **647**   FAT: **49g**   CARBOHYDRATES: **33g**   FIBER: **4g**   SUGARS: **15g**   PROTEIN: **23g**

AMP UP THE FAT AND PROTEIN:

 ADD MORE CHICKEN AND DRIZZLE WITH MORE AVOCADO OIL.

GF **EF**

You will love this satisfying Caesar salad with roasted broccoli, grilled chicken, and golden Parmesan crisps. The crisps add a perfect crunchy element to the salad so you won't miss the croutons.

CHICKEN AND BROCCOLI CAESAR SALAD

SERVES: 2   **PREP: 20 MINUTES**   **COOK: 30 MINUTES**

4 slices bacon

8oz (226g) broccoli florets

1 tsp avocado oil

Sea salt and freshly ground black pepper, to taste

8oz (226g) boneless skinless chicken breast

6 cups coarsely chopped romaine lettuce (about 2 medium romaine hearts)

¼ cup thinly sliced scallions

Caesar dressing:

⅓ cup (0.3oz/9g) finely grated fresh Parmesan cheese

3 tbsp avocado oil

3 tbsp fresh lemon juice

2 tsp Dijon mustard

2 garlic cloves

Sea salt and freshly ground black pepper, to taste

Parmesan crisps:

½ cup (0.5oz/14g) finely grated fresh Parmesan cheese (microplane recommended; not prepackaged shreds)

1 Make the Caesar dressing. In small food processor or blender, process all of the ingredients until smooth. Refrigerate until ready to use.

2 Make the crisps. Preheat the oven to 375°F (190°C). Line a baking sheet with parchment paper. Place 6 (2-tablespoon) mounds of Parmesan on the baking sheet about 2 inches (5cm) apart. Spread each mound into a 3-inch (7.5cm) circle. Bake for 5 to 7 minutes or until lightly browned and bubbling. Let stand on the baking sheet for a minute, and then carefully remove to a plate or board to cool.

3 Increase the oven temperature to 400°F (200°C). Place a greased wire rack on the same baking sheet. Arrange the bacon in a single layer at one end of the rack.

4 In a medium bowl, toss the broccoli with the oil, and sprinkle with salt and pepper. Arrange the broccoli in a single layer at the other end of the rack. Cook for 20 minutes or until the bacon is cooked and the broccoli is tender-crisp.

5 While the broccoli and bacon are cooking, preheat a grill or a grill pan to medium-high. Sprinkle the chicken with salt and pepper. Cook the chicken on the greased grill for 5 to 7 minutes on each side or until thoroughly cooked.

6 Slice the chicken and chop the bacon. Place the romaine in two serving bowls, and top with the chicken, broccoli, bacon, and scallions. Drizzle with the dressing. Break up the Parmesan crisps and add them to the salad. Serve immediately.

NUTRITION PER SERVING

CALORIES: **535**   FAT: **38g**   CARBOHYDRATES: **16g**   FIBER: **6g**   SUGARS: **5g**   PROTEIN: **36g**

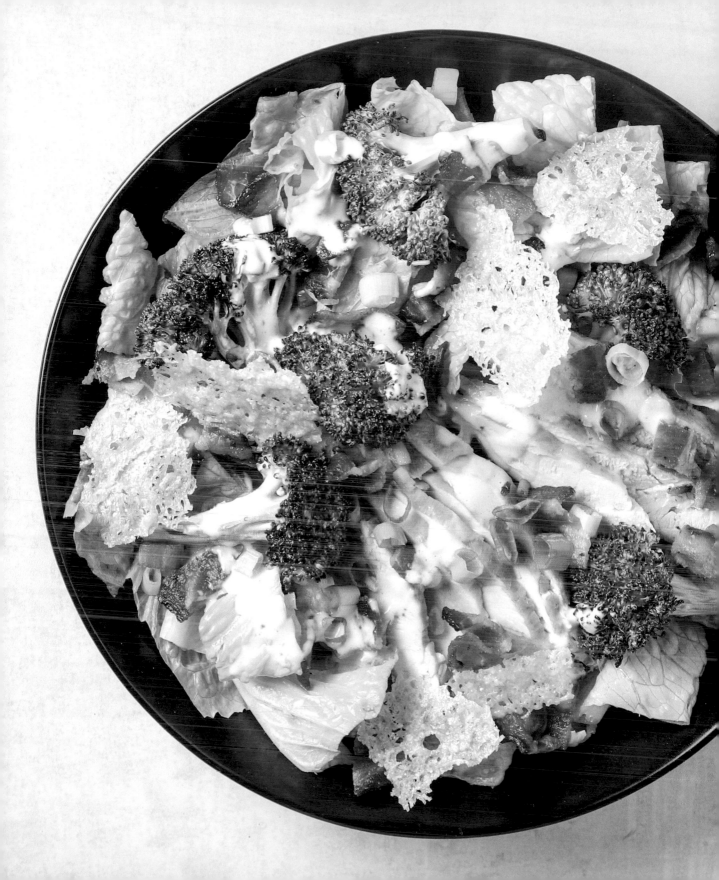

This fresh and summery salad is best when strawberries and asparagus are at their peak. Switch out the nuts or cheese to any variety you prefer. Chopped, roasted chicken is a delicious addition.

STRAWBERRY GOAT CHEESE SALAD WITH POPPY SEED DRESSING

✖ SERVES: **1**　　　🕐 PREP: **10 MINUTES**　　　🔥 COOK: **NONE**

4 cups spring mix

1 small cucumber

8 asparagus spears, trimmed of woody ends

1 cup (152g) sliced strawberries (hulled)

2 tbsp chopped pecans

1 slice cooked bacon, diced (about 2 tbsp)

1 mandarin orange, segmented

1 oz (28g) creamy goat cheese, broken into small pieces

Lemon poppy seed dressing:

1½ tbsp mayonnaise

1 tbsp fresh lemon juice

Pinch of stevia or granulated monk fruit sweetener (optional)

1 tsp poppy seeds

½ tsp Dijon mustard

Sea salt and freshly ground black pepper, to taste

1 Make the lemon poppy seed dressing. In a small bowl, whisk together all of the ingredients.

2 In a shallow serving bowl, arrange the spring mix. Using a vegetable peeler, peel long strips of the cucumber and long strips of the asparagus onto the spring mix.

3 Add the strawberries, pecans, bacon, mandarin segments, and goat cheese. Drizzle with the dressing. Toss gently to combine, and serve immediately.

NUTRITION PER SERVING

CALORIES: **609**　FAT: **41g**　CARBOHYDRATES: **40g**　FIBER: **10g**　SUGARS: **21g**　PROTEIN: **10g**

This is a crunchy, fresh salad with a creamy homemade ranch dressing. Try making your own mayonnaise (page 209) for the most delicious result. You will need 1½ cups of chopped, cooked chicken for this recipe, such as leftovers from the Roasted Herb Chicken and Gravy (page 178).

CHICKEN RANCH CHOP SALAD

✖ SERVES: **2**   🕐 PREP: **15 MINUTES**   🔥 COOK: **NONE**

4 cups chopped or shredded romaine lettuce

1½ cups chopped cooked chicken

1 cup chopped celery

¼ cup thinly sliced scallions

1 green bell pepper, seeds and membranes removed, chopped

¼ cup walnuts, toasted and chopped

Ranch dressing:

2 tbsp mayonnaise

2 tbsp sour cream

2 tbsp fresh lemon juice

1 tbsp water

1 tbsp finely chopped dill

1 tbsp finely chopped flat-leaf parsley

½ tsp onion powder

½ tsp garlic powder

Sea salt and freshly ground black pepper, to taste

1 Make the ranch dressing. In a small bowl, whisk together all of the ingredients until well combined.

2 In two shallow serving bowls, arrange the romaine, chicken, celery, scallions, bell pepper, and walnuts. Drizzle with the dressing, and toss to combine. Serve immediately.

NUTRITION PER SERVING

CALORIES: **433**   FAT: **27g**   CARBOHYDRATES: **12g**   FIBER: **5g**   SUGARS: **5g**   PROTEIN: **38g**

You will love all the crunch from the radishes, cucumber, and lettuce. This cobb salad is topped with roasted beef and tomato, and then it's drizzled with a smoky, hot ranch dressing. This is a good way to use leftover roast beef, or purchase deli-sliced roasted beef from the store. Make sure to leave the fat on!

BEEF COBB SALAD WITH CHIPOTLE RANCH DRESSING

SERVES: 2 **PREP: 20 MINUTES** **COOK: NONE**

2 cups shredded romaine lettuce

4oz (113g) grape tomatoes, halved

2 large hard-boiled eggs, peeled

8oz (226g) deli-sliced roast beef or shredded roasted chicken

½ cup sliced cucumber

½ cup sliced radish

2 slices red onion, separated into rings

¼ cup grated white Cheddar cheese

Sliced avocado (optional), for serving

Chipotle ranch dressing:

3 tbsp chopped cilantro

2 tbsp mayonnaise

2 tbsp sour cream

2 tbsp fresh lemon juice

1 tbsp olive oil

1 tbsp water

1 chipotle pepper in adobo sauce

1 tbsp adobo sauce (from the peppers)

½ tsp garlic powder

Sea salt and freshly ground black pepper, to taste

1 Make the chipotle ranch dressing. In a small bowl, whisk together all of the dressing ingredients until well combined.

2 On two individual plates or one serving platter, arrange the romaine, tomatoes, eggs, beef, cucumber, radishes, onion, and Cheddar. Drizzle with the dressing and top with sliced avocado (if using). Serve immediately.

NUTRITION PER SERVING

CALORIES: **526**   FAT: **37g**   CARBOHYDRATES: **12g**   FIBER: **3g**   SUGARS: **5g**   PROTEIN: **38g**

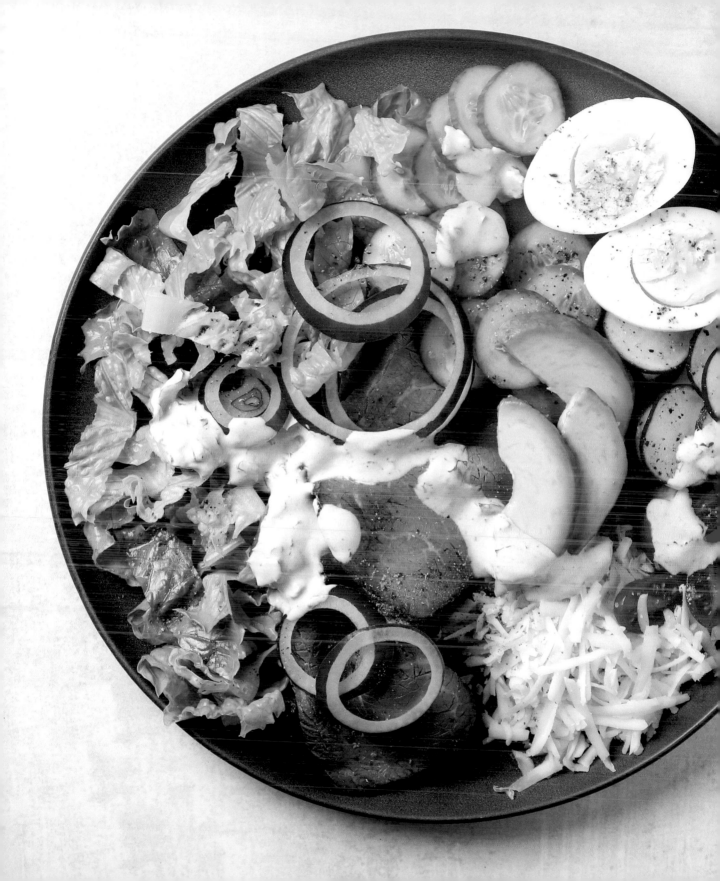

Baby spinach leaves make the perfect base for chicken, pecans, juicy strawberries, asparagus, and creamy goat cheese. The salad is then drizzled with a balsamic, lemon, and mustard vinaigrette.

CHICKEN AND GOAT CHEESE SALAD

SERVES: **2**   PREP: **15 MINUTES**   COOK: **NONE**

4 cups baby spinach leaves

6oz (170g) shredded chicken

½ cup sliced strawberries (hulled)

¼ cup coarsely chopped pecans, toasted

8 asparagus spears, trimmed of woody ends

2oz (67g) creamy goat cheese, broken into small pieces

Mustard balsamic vinaigrette:

2 tbsp olive oil

1 tbsp balsamic vinegar

1 tbsp fresh lemon juice

1 tsp Dijon mustard

¼ tsp garlic powder

Sea salt and freshly ground black pepper, to taste

1 Make the mustard balsamic vinaigrette. In a small bowl, whisk together all of the ingredients until well combined.

2 In two serving bowls, arrange the spinach leaves. Top with the chicken, strawberries, and pecans. Using a vegetable peeler, peel long strips of the asparagus onto the salad.

3 Drizzle the salad with dressing. Top with the goat cheese and serve immediately.

NUTRITION PER SERVING

CALORIES: **474**   FAT: **35g**   CARBOHYDRATES: **11g**   FIBER: **5g**   SUGARS: **6g**   PROTEIN: **32g**

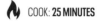
Kids and adults will love this salad—chicken tenders, coated in almond flour, Parmesan, and lemon pepper seasoning, and baked until golden! The tenders are served on a bed of greens and drizzled with a mustard and Parmesan dressing.

ALMOND AND PARMESAN CHICKEN SALAD

SERVES: 3   **PREP: 26 MINUTES**   **COOK: 25 MINUTES**

9 chicken tenderloins

2 large eggs

1 cup blanched almond flour

½ cup (0.5oz/14g) finely grated fresh Parmesan cheese

1 tsp lemon pepper seasoning

1 tsp garlic powder

Sea salt, to taste

Olive oil cooking spray (optional)

3 artisan lettuce hearts, halved lengthwise, stems removed, leaves separated and chopped (about 5 cups chopped)

1½ cups thinly sliced celery

3 tbsp sliced almonds, toasted

Sliced Persian cucumbers (optional), for serving

Parmesan dressing:

½ cup (0.5oz/14g) finely grated fresh Parmesan cheese

3 tbsp avocado oil

2 tbsp fresh lemon juice

2 tbsp water

2 tsp spicy brown mustard

¼ tsp garlic powder

1 Make the Parmesan dressing. In a small blender or food processor, process all of the ingredients until smooth and creamy, adding an extra tablespoon water if the dressing is too thick.

2 Preheat the oven to 375°F (190°C). Line a baking sheet with parchment paper.

3 Using a small, sharp knife, carefully remove and discard the white tendon from under each tenderloin. (This is optional, but the tendon can be chewy if left. Sometimes the tendon is already removed when purchased.)

4 In a shallow bowl, whisk the eggs until they are slightly frothy. In a separate shallow bowl, place the almond flour, Parmesan, lemon pepper seasoning, garlic powder, and salt. Whisk or stir to combine.

5 Dip each tenderloin into the egg, and then coat in the almond flour mixture, pressing the chicken into the almond mixture. Place in a single layer on the baking sheet. Spray the tenderloins with olive oil spray (if using) to help them crisp up.

6 Bake for 23 to 25 minutes, turning halfway through cooking, or until the chicken is golden and cooked. Cut crosswise into slices to serve.

7 On three serving plates, arrange the lettuce and celery. Arrange the chicken on top. Drizzle with the dressing, sprinkle with the almonds, and top with sliced cucumber (if using). Serve immediately.

NUTRITION PER SERVING

CALORIES: **582**   FAT: **47g**   CARBOHYDRATES: **14g**   FIBER: **6g**   SUGARS: **3g**   PROTEIN: **39g**

AMP UP THE FAT AND PROTEIN:

ADD EXTRA CASHEWS OR SLICED AVOCADO.

GF EF DF

With bright flavors reminiscent of Southeast Asia, this salad is loaded with fresh veggies, fresh herbs, and a creamy satay dressing.

THAI BEEF SALAD WITH SATAY DRESSING

SERVES: 2   **PREP: 15 MINUTES**   **COOK: 10 MINUTES**

10oz (283g) New York strip steak (sirloin)

1 tsp avocado oil

Sea salt and freshly ground black pepper, to taste

3 cups shredded romaine lettuce

½ cup shredded red cabbage

½ cup chopped cucumber

¼ cup coarsely chopped mint leaves

¼ cup coarsely chopped cilantro

Peanuts (optional), toasted and chopped, for garnish

Thinly sliced red onion (optional), for garnish

Satay dressing:

3 tbsp fresh lime juice

3 tbsp natural peanut butter

2 tbsp water

1-2 tbsp coconut aminos

1 tbsp avocado oil

1 tsp sesame oil

1 tsp sriracha sauce

½ tsp garlic powder

1 Make the satay dressing. In a small bowl, whisk together all of the ingredients until smooth. Set aside.

2 Heat a grill pan or grill to medium-high. Rub the steak with the oil and season with salt and pepper. Cook the steak for 5 minutes on each side or until cooked as desired. Transfer to a cutting board. Cover with foil and let rest for 10 minutes. Cut against the grain into thin slices.

3 In two serving bowls, arrange the romaine, cabbage, and cucumber. Drizzle with a spoonful of dressing. Top with steak strips, mint, and cilantro. Drizzle with the remaining dressing. Top with peanuts and onion slices (if using), and serve immediately.

NUTRITION PER SERVING

CALORIES: **446**   FAT: **28g**   CARBOHYDRATES: **13g**   FIBER: **3g**   SUGARS: **4g**   PROTEIN: **37g**

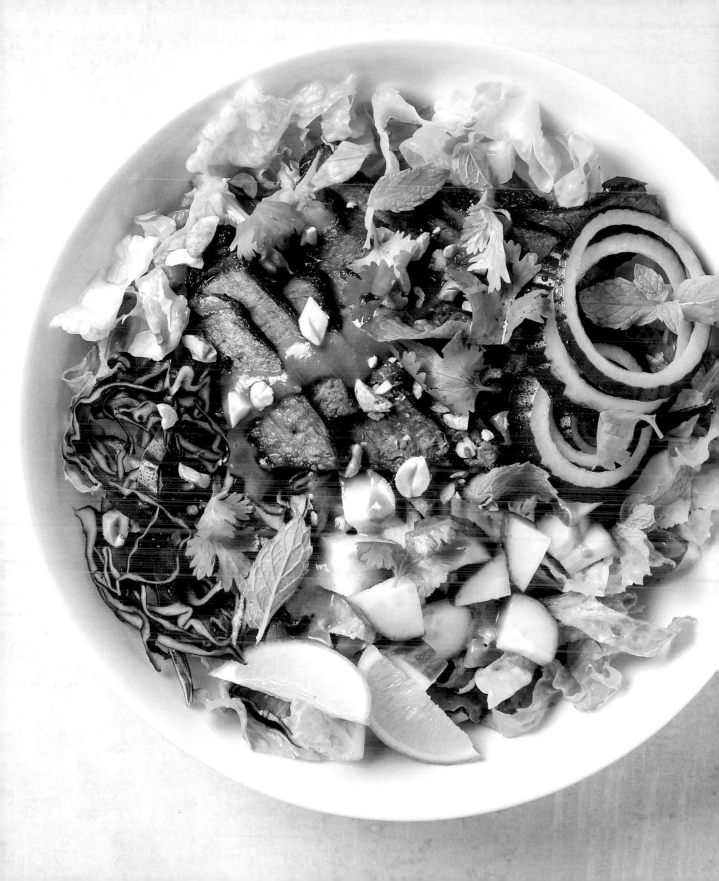

10

ONE-PAN ENTRÉES + PROTEIN HEADLINERS

Browned pork is flavored with ginger, garlic, and mint and then spooned into lettuce cups and topped with a spicy cucumber salad and avocado. This is a great sharing meal—place the lettuce, pork, and salad on a platter, and let everyone help themselves.

PORK LETTUCE WRAPS WITH SPICY CUCUMBER SALAD

SERVES: **4**   PREP: **20 MINUTES**   COOK: **10 MINUTES**

1 head butter lettuce

1 tbsp avocado oil

20oz (567g) ground pork or turkey

2 tbsp finely grated ginger

3 garlic cloves, minced

2 tbsp coconut aminos

1 tbsp fresh lime juice

⅓ cup coarsely chopped mint leaves, plus extra leaves for serving

1 avocado, chopped

Cashews (optional), toasted and chopped, for serving

Spicy cucumber salad:

2 tbsp coconut aminos

2 tbsp fresh lime juice

1 English cucumber, sliced

½ cup sliced radishes (about 5 radishes)

¼ small red onion, thinly sliced

2 small red chilies, or more to taste

1 Make the spicy cucumber salad. In a medium bowl, combine all of the ingredients. Cover and refrigerate until ready to serve.

2 Trim and discard the stem from the head of lettuce. Separate the leaves and place into a large bowl of cool water. Let stand.

3 In a large skillet, heat the oil over medium-high heat. Add the pork. Cook, breaking up any large pieces, for 8 to 10 minutes or until browned.

4 Add the ginger and garlic. Cook, stirring constantly, for 1 minute or until fragrant. Remove from the heat.

5 Add the coconut aminos, lime juice, and mint. Stir until combined.

6 Remove the lettuce from the water and shake off any excess. Gently pat dry with paper towels.

7 Arrange the lettuce on a plate. Divide the pork among the lettuce cups. Using a slotted spoon, drain any excess dressing from the salad and spoon into the lettuce cups. Top with the avocado. Sprinkle with extra mint leaves and cashews (if using). Serve immediately.

NUTRITION PER SERVING

CALORIES: **533**   FAT: **41g**   CARBOHYDRATES: **15g**   FIBER: **5g**   SUGARS: **3g**   PROTEIN: **27g**

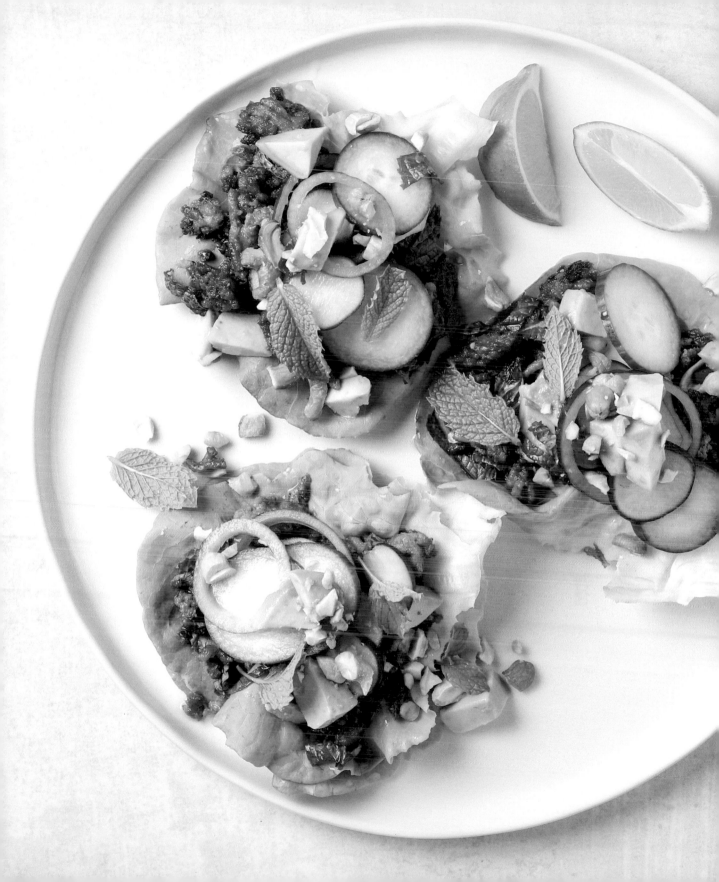

AMP UP THE FAT AND PROTEIN:

 ADD EXTRA BEEF.

GF **DF** **EF**

Freshly ground black pepper, fresh ginger, and garlic give this stir-fry bold flavor, and the broccoli adds crisp texture. Have all of your ingredients prepped and ready at the start—this dish comes together quickly!

PEPPERY GINGER BEEF AND BROCCOLI STIR-FRY

✖️ SERVES: **2**   🕐 PREP: **15 MINUTES**   🔥 COOK: **7 MINUTES**

½ cup beef broth

3 tbsp coconut aminos

1 tbsp sriracha sauce

⅛ tsp xanthan gum

2 tbsp avocado oil

10oz (283g) sirloin beef steak (such as New York strip), thinly sliced against the grain

½–1 tsp freshly ground black pepper

2 garlic cloves, sliced

1in (2.5cm) piece fresh ginger, julienned

5oz (142g) broccoli florets (about 2 cups)

Whole almonds (optional), toasted, for serving

1 In a small bowl or liquid measuring cup, combine the broth, coconut aminos, sriracha, and xanthan gum. Set aside.

2 In a large wok or skillet, heat the oil over high heat. Add the beef. Stir-fry for 2 minutes or until the beef has browned. Remove the beef from the pan.

3 Add the pepper to taste, garlic, and ginger. Stir-fry for 20 seconds or until fragrant.

4 Add the broccoli and stir-fry for 2 minutes or until bright green. Stir the broth mixture and add to the wok. Stir-fry until the broccoli is tender-crisp, about 4 minutes.

5 Add the beef. Stir-fry until combined and hot. Serve immediately sprinkled with almonds (if using).

NUTRITION PER SERVING

CALORIES: **411**   FAT: **24g**   CARBOHYDRATES: **13g**   FIBER: **3g**   SUGARS: **1g**   PROTEIN: **36g**

Use red or green cabbage in this recipe—or both!—for a colorful, crisp, and satisfying meal. Be sure to have all of your ingredients ready to go before you start cooking.

PORK, PEPPER, AND CABBAGE STIR-FRY

SERVES: **2**   PREP: **20 MINUTES**   COOK. **8 MINUTES**

¼ cup chicken broth

3 tbsp coconut aminos

1 tsp sesame oil

1 tsp stevia or granulated monk fruit sweetener (optional)

1 tsp freshly ground black pepper

1 tbsp avocado oil

10oz (281g) pork tenderloin, thinly sliced into strips

2 garlic cloves, sliced

1 tbsp finely grated ginger

1 large green bell pepper, seeds and membranes removed, sliced

1½ cups shredded red cabbage

½ cup thinly sliced celery

2 small red chilies, thinly sliced

5 scallions, trimmed and cut into 1-in (2.5cm) lengths

½ cup slivered or sliced almonds, toasted

1 In a small bowl or liquid measuring cup, combine the broth, coconut aminos, sesame oil, stevia (if using), and black pepper. Set aside.

2 In a large wok or skillet, heat the oil over medium-high heat. Add the pork and stir-fry for 3 minutes or until the pork is no longer pink.

3 Add the garlic and ginger and stir-fry for 30 seconds or until fragrant. Add the green pepper and stir-fry for 2 minutes or until starting to soften.

4 Add the cabbage and celery. Stir-fry for 2 minutes or until the cabbage is starting to soften but still crisp.

5 Stir the broth mixture and add to the wok, along with the red chilies and scallions. Stir-fry for 30 seconds or until combined and the sauce is hot. Remove from the heat.

6 Add the almonds and toss to combine. Serve immediately.

NUTRITION PER SERVING

CALORIES: **493**   FAT: **28g**   CARBOHYDRATES: **22g**   FIBER: **7g**   SUGARS: **6g**   PROTEIN: **40g**

This hearty roasted chicken, with its crispy, herby skin and creamy gravy, is loved by many. Serve with Cheesy Mashed Cauliflower (page 201) and Almond Thyme Green Beans (page 200) for the ultimate comfort meal.

ROASTED HERB CHICKEN AND GRAVY

SERVES: 4   **PREP: 20 MINUTES**   **COOK: 1 HOUR 20 MINUTES**

Roasted chicken:

3lb (1.3kg) whole chicken

1-2 tbsp softened butter

3 tbsp chopped flat-leaf parsley

2 tsp chopped rosemary

1 tsp chopped thyme or sage

1 tsp garlic powder

Sea salt and freshly ground black pepper, to taste

Gravy:

3 tbsp pan drippings

2½ cups chicken broth

½ tsp freshly ground black pepper

1 tsp Worcestershire sauce or coconut aminos

Sea salt, to taste

¾ tsp xanthan gum

1 Grease a wire rack and place it in an oven-safe roasting pan or baking dish. Preheat the oven to 375°F (190°C). Prepare the chicken. If it isn't already spatchcocked, turn the chicken onto its breast. Using poultry scissors or a sharp filleting or chef's knife, cut alongside both sides of the backbone to remove it. Turn the chicken breast-side up. Turn the wings in and tuck the tips behind the chicken. Carefully run your fingers underneath the skin of the chicken to loosen it from the flesh.

2 In a small bowl, use a fork to combine the butter, parsley, rosemary, thyme, garlic powder, salt, and pepper.

3 Reserve about ½ tablespoon butter mixture and spread the rest evenly between the skin and the flesh of the breast, thighs, and drumsticks.

4 Place the chicken breast-side up on the prepared rack. Spread the remaining butter over the skin of the chicken. Season with salt and pepper. Roast, uncovered, for about 1 hour 15 minutes or until the juices run clear when the chicken is pierced around the thigh bone or a thermometer reads 165°F (74°C) when inserted into the thickest part of the thigh. Cover loosely with foil and let stand for 5 minutes. Chop or carve the chicken to serve.

5 Make the gravy. Reserve 3 tablespoons of the pan drippings and discard any remaining. In the same pan, whisk together the drippings, broth, pepper, Worcestershire sauce, and salt, and bring to a boil. Whisk in the xanthan gum. Let simmer for 5 minutes or until thickened. Add extra broth or water if the gravy is too thick. Serve immediately with the chicken.

NUTRITION PER SERVING (for ¼ of the chicken and ½ cup gravy)

CALORIES: **220**   FAT: **10g**   CARBOHYDRATES: **1g**   FIBER: **0g**   SUGARS: **1g**   PROTEIN: **30g**

You can request a butcher to spatchcock the chicken for you, or follow the instructions to do it yourself.

AMP UP THE FAT AND PROTEIN: **PREPARE EXTRA WRAPPED SHRIMP.**

GF DF EF

Broccoli, sweet bell peppers, garlic, and a touch of heat—this lemony, quick, and fully satisfying dinner is all roasted on one pan, making for easy clean-up.

ONE-PAN PROSCIUTTO-WRAPPED SHRIMP AND BROCCOLI

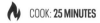

SERVES: **2**   PREP: **15 MINUTES**   COOK: **25 MINUTES**

6 small bell peppers (any colors), halved, seeds and membranes removed

16oz (487g) broccoli, trimmed and cut into florets

1 lemon, sliced, plus extra wedges for serving

2 tbsp olive oil, divided

Sea salt and freshly ground black pepper, to taste

8 slices prosciutto, halved lengthwise

16 large raw shrimp, peeled and deveined, tails intact

2 garlic cloves, sliced

½ tsp crushed red pepper

2 tbsp chopped flat-leaf parsley

6 tbsp (42g) sliced almonds, toasted

1 Preheat the oven to 400°F (200°F). Line a baking sheet with parchment paper.

2 On the baking sheet, toss together bell pepper halves, broccoli, lemon slices, 1 tablespoon oil, salt, and pepper. Roast for 7 minutes.

3 Wrap half a slice of prosciutto around each shrimp. Add the wrapped shrimp to the partially cooked pepper and broccoli mixture. Drizzle with the remaining 1 tablespoon oil. Add the garlic and crushed red pepper. Toss to combine. Bake for 15 minutes or until the shrimp are just cooked and the vegetables are tender-crisp.

4 Add the parsley. Toss to combine. Sprinkle with almonds and serve immediately with lemon wedges.

NUTRITION PER SERVING

CALORIES: **512**   FAT: **36g**   CARBOHYDRATES: **23g**   FIBER: **11g**   SUGARS: **6g**   PROTEIN: **28g**

This warm, comforting recipe cooks in one skillet. It's a great way to use up vegetables lurking in the fridge. For example, you could switch the eggplant for zucchini and add bell peppers for a variation.

SPICY CHICKEN AND EGGPLANT

✕ SERVES: **4**   🕐 PREP: **20 MINUTES**   🔥 COOK: **50 MINUTES**

4 bone-in chicken thighs

1 tbsp olive oil

1 medium red onion, sliced

4 garlic cloves, minced

3 tbsp tomato paste

1 (14oz/398ml) can diced
  tomatoes, undrained

1½ cups chicken broth

1-2 tsp crushed red pepper

1lb (450g) eggplant, chopped

Sea salt and freshly ground
  black pepper, to taste

⅓ cup pitted Kalamata olives

⅓ cup chopped flat-leaf parsley

1 tbsp capers

2 tbsp fresh lemon juice

16oz (454g) steamed broccoli
  (optional), for serving

1 Remove and discard the skin from the chicken. In a large skillet or Dutch oven, heat the oil over medium-high heat. Add the chicken and cook for 5 minutes on each side or until golden brown. Remove from the skillet.

2 Add the onion to the skillet. Cook, stirring occasionally, for 5 minutes or until the onion has softened. Add the garlic and tomato paste. Cook, stirring, until fragrant, about 30 seconds.

3 Add the tomatoes with their juices, broth, crushed red pepper to taste, eggplant, salt, and pepper. Stir to combine.

4 Return the chicken to the skillet. Bring to a boil. Cover and reduce the heat to medium-low. Cook for 20 minutes, stirring and turning the chicken once during the cook time. Uncover and cook for 15 minutes more, turning the chicken once, until the chicken is cooked and the sauce has thickened.

5 Add the olives, parsley, capers, and lemon juice. Stir to combine. Cook, uncovered, for 3 minutes or until the olives are hot. Serve immediately with steamed broccoli (if using).

NUTRITION PER SERVING (excluding broccoli)

CALORIES: **456**   FAT: **30g**   CARBOHYDRATES: **22g**   FIBER: **7g**   SUGARS: **11g**   PROTEIN: **28g**

AMP UP THE FAT AND PROTEIN:

 ADD TOASTED NUTS, SUCH AS CASHEWS OR ALMONDS.

GF EF V

This wholesome, creamy, and delicious curry comes together easily. Leftovers are even more flavorful the next day and will keep up to 5 days in a sealed container in the refrigerator.

QUICK AND EASY VEGETABLE CURRY

🍴 SERVES: **4**   🕐 PREP: **20 MINUTES**   🔥 COOK: **20 MINUTES**

1 tbsp butter

1 cup diced yellow onion

4 garlic cloves, minced

1 tbsp finely grated fresh ginger

¼ cup mild or medium curry paste (such as any flavor of Patak's Curry Paste), or to taste

1 (14oz/398ml) can full-fat coconut milk

2 cups vegetable broth

1 cauliflower head (about 28oz/800g whole), trimmed and cut into florets

1 eggplant (about 1lb/450g), trimmed, halved, and thickly sliced

1 small bunch kale, stems removed, leaves coarsely chopped (about 5 heaped cups)

½ cup plain full-fat yogurt, plus extra for serving

⅓ cup coarsely chopped cilantro, plus extra for serving

2 tbsp fresh lemon juice

Sea salt and freshly ground black pepper, to taste

1 In a large pot or Dutch oven, melt the butter over medium heat. Add the onion, garlic, and ginger, and cook, stirring occasionally, for 5 minutes or until the onion is softened.

2 Add the curry paste to taste and cook for 1 minute, or until fragrant. Stir in the coconut milk and broth.

3 Add the cauliflower and stir to coat in the curry mixture. Cover, increase the heat to high, and bring to a boil. Reduce the heat to medium and cook, covered, for 5 minutes. Add the eggplant and cook, covered, for 7 to 10 minutes or until softened.

4 Add the kale and gently stir to combine. Cover and cook for 2 to 3 minutes or until the kale is wilted and bright green.

5 Add the yogurt, cilantro, and lemon juice, and gently stir to combine. Taste and season with salt and pepper. Serve individual portions with extra yogurt and cilantro, if desired.

NUTRITION PER SERVING

CALORIES: **357**   FAT: **22g**   CARBOHYDRATES: **28g**   FIBER: **8g**   SUGARS: **12g**   PROTEIN: **9g**

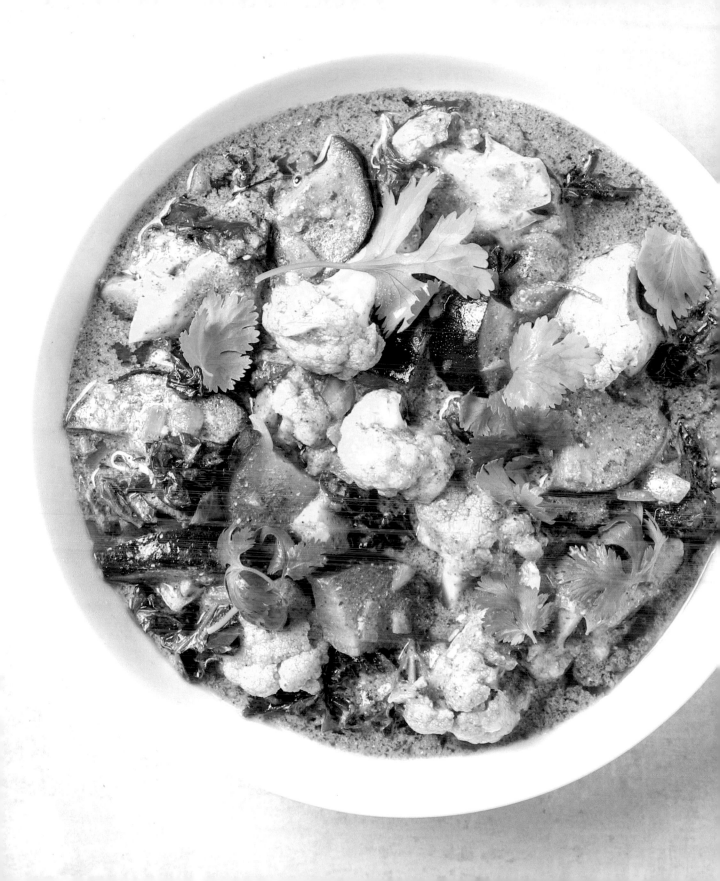

AMP UP THE FAT AND PROTEIN:

 SERVE WITH SLICED AVOCADO.

GF

The pico de gallo adds a nice level of acidity to cut the richness of this Mexican-inspired meatloaf. Serve with Spanish Cauliflower Rice (page 204). Any leftover meatloaf can be added to a salad or served with steamed vegetables for tomorrow's evening meal. Reserve some of the pico de gallo for Mexican Omelets (page 148).

MEXICAN MEATLOAF

✖️ SERVES: **5**   🕐 PREP: **20 MINUTES**   🔥 COOK: **50 MINUTES**

1 large egg

1lb (450g) ground beef (20% fat)

4oz (113g) ground pork

¾ cup blanched almond flour

½ cup diced white onion

½ cup grated pepper jack cheese

⅓ cup finely chopped cilantro

2 garlic cloves, minced

1 tbsp smoked paprika or chipotle powder

1 tbsp chili powder

1 tsp sea salt

2 tbsp sugar-free ketchup

Pico de gallo:

3 vine-ripened tomatoes (1lb/454g), diced

½ cup diced white onion

⅓ cup chopped cilantro leaves and stems

1 jalapeño, diced

3 tbsp fresh lime juice

Sea salt and freshly ground black pepper, to taste

1 Preheat the oven to 375°F (190°C). Line a baking sheet with parchment paper.

2 In a medium bowl, whisk the egg. Add the beef, pork, almond flour, onion, cheese, cilantro, garlic, paprika, chili powder, and salt. Mix with your hands until well combined.

3 Lay a sheet of parchment paper on the counter. Turn the beef mixture out onto the parchment. Press the mixture into a 10 x 12-inch (25 x 30cm) rectangle. Roll up (Swiss roll style) from one short side, using the paper as a guide. Place on the baking sheet, seam-side down.

4 Bake for 30 minutes. Remove from the oven and carefully pour off and discard any fat, if necessary. Brush the loaf with the ketchup. Bake for 20 minutes or until firm and a meat thermometer inserted in the center reads 160°F (71°C). Cover loosely with foil and let stand for 10 minutes before cutting into 10 slices (about 1in/2.5cm thick).

5 While the meatloaf is baking, make the pico de gallo. In a small bowl, combine all of the ingredients. Serve with the meatloaf.

NUTRITION PER SERVING (2 slices of meatloaf)

CALORIES: **477**   FAT: **36g**   CARBOHYDRATES: **12g**   FIBER: **4g**   SUGARS: **4g**   PROTEIN: **28g**

Garlic and herb butter portobello mushrooms are topped with melted Swiss cheese, grilled until tender, and served on low-carb Sesame Seed Buns (page 206). For a quick and easy side, serve with crunchy slaw (page 195).

MUSHROOM AND SWISS "BURGERS"

SERVES: **2**   PREP: **15 MINUTES**   COOK: **10 MINUTES**

2 tbsp softened butter

2 tbsp chopped flat-leaf parsley

1 tbsp whole-grain mustard, plus extra for serving

2 garlic cloves, minced

½ tsp sweet or smoked paprika

Sea salt and freshly ground black pepper, to taste

2 portobello mushrooms

2 slices Swiss cheese

2 Sesame Seed Buns (page 206), split

Lettuce, tomato slices, red onion slices, and avocado slices (optional), for serving

1 In a small bowl, combine the butter, parsley, mustard, garlic, paprika, salt, and pepper.

2 Grease and preheat a grill or a grill pan to medium-high. Cook the mushrooms cap-side down on the greased grill for 5 minutes or until grill marks appear. Turn the mushrooms over. Divide the butter mixture into the caps. Cook for 3 to 5 minutes or until the butter is melted and the mushrooms are cooked. (The cook time may vary depending on the size of the mushrooms.) Top each mushroom (on the gill side) with cheese.

3 On the same grill, toast the buns for 2 to 3 minutes or until grill marks appear.

4 Spread the bottom of the buns with extra mustard. Top the buns with lettuce, tomato, and onion (if using). Place the cooked mushrooms on top, and finally add avocado slices (if using). Replace the bun tops and serve.

NUTRITION PER SERVING (excluding the toppings)

CALORIES: **506**   FAT: **38g**   CARBOHYDRATES: **29g**   FIBER: **17g**   SUGARS: **4g**   PROTEIN: **19g**

This dish is loaded with crisp vegetables and succulent shrimp. It uses cauliflower instead of rice to keep the carbs low and the fiber high. Use fresh cauliflower and blitz it in a food processor, or use store-bought riced cauliflower, found in the produce or freezer sections of most grocery stores.

SHRIMP FRIED CAULIFLOWER RICE

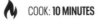

🍴 SERVES: **3**   🕐 PREP: **20 MINUTES**   🔥 COOK: **10 MINUTES**

1 tbsp avocado oil

3 large eggs

4 slices bacon, diced

3 garlic cloves, minced

2 tbsp finely chopped fresh ginger

12oz (346g) raw large shrimp, peeled and deveined

4oz (113g) snow peas, trimmed

8oz (226g) asparagus, trimmed of woody ends and cut into 1-in (2.5cm) pieces

3 tbsp coconut aminos

1 tsp crushed red pepper

4 cups cauliflower rice (frozen and thawed, or fresh)

⅓ cup coarsely chopped cilantro, plus extra for garnish

⅓ cup thinly sliced scallions, plus extra for garnish

1. In a large wok or skillet, heat the oil over high heat. In a small bowl, whisk the eggs until well combined.

2. When the oil is hot, add the beaten eggs, turning the wok to coat the bottom. Reduce the heat to medium. Cook for about 3 minutes or until set, swirling the wok and lifting the omelet to allow the uncooked egg to flow underneath. When the egg is almost set, fold the omelet over, loosely rolling it up. Transfer to a small cutting board and cut into ribbons. Set aside.

3. Add the bacon to the wok. Cook over medium-high heat, stirring occasionally, for 5 minutes or until browned and starting to crisp. Remove the bacon from the wok to a paper towel–lined plate. Drain and discard all but 1 tablespoon fat from the wok.

4. Heat the wok again with the tablespoon of bacon fat over medium-high heat. Add the garlic, ginger, and shrimp, and stir-fry for 2 minutes or until the shrimp are starting to change color.

5. Add the cooked bacon, snow peas, and asparagus. Stir-fry over high heat until the vegetables are tender-crisp. Add the coconut aminos and red pepper flakes. Stir-fry until combined.

6. Add the cauliflower rice and cilantro. Stir-fry for 1 minute or until the cauliflower is hot. Add the scallions and stir-fry until just combined. Garnish with extra cilantro and scallions, and serve immediately.

NUTRITION PER SERVING

CALORIES: **495**   FAT: **28g**   CARBOHYDRATES: **23g**   FIBER: **7g**   SUGARS: **8g**   PROTEIN: **40g**

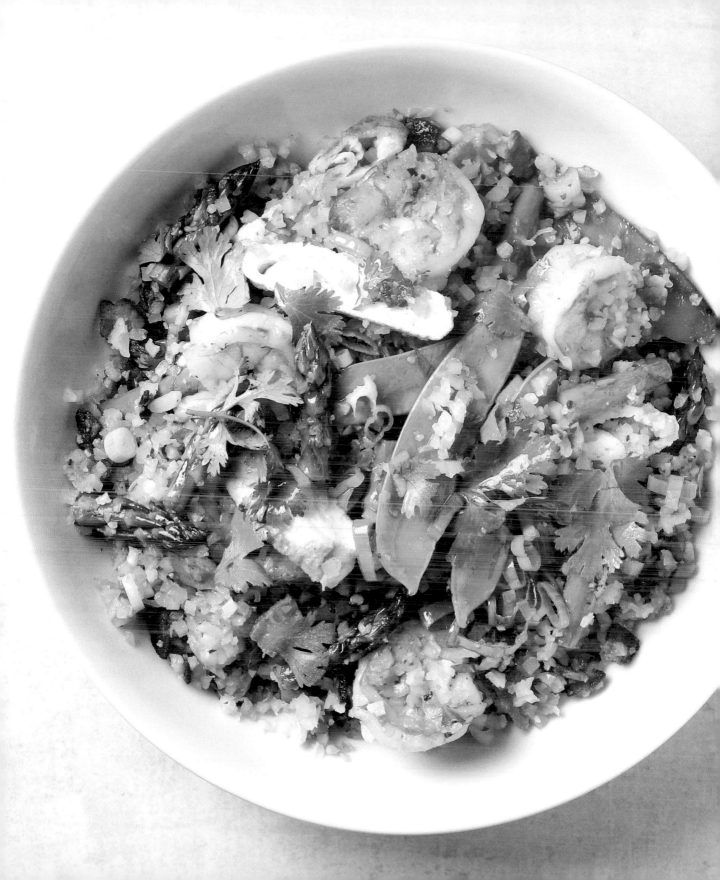

AMP UP THE FAT AND PROTEIN:
SERVE WITH CHEESY MASHED CAULIFLOWER (PAGE 201).

GF

Tender salmon is topped with a low-carb breadcrumb, Parmesan, and fresh herb topping and then baked and served on a bed of just-wilted spinach. Feel free to use whatever fresh herb combination you prefer—tarragon, dill, chives, parsley, thyme, and rosemary all will work, or simply use flat-leaf parsley.

PARMESAN HERB CRUSTED SALMON WITH SAUTÉED SPINACH

SERVES: **2**   PREP: **20 MINUTES**   COOK: **15 MINUTES**

8oz (225g) salmon fillet

1 large egg white

½ cup low-carb breadcrumbs (about half of a Sesame Seed Bun, page 206, processed; see the tip)

⅓ cup (0.3oz/9g) finely grated fresh Parmesan cheese

3 tbsp chopped flat-leaf parsley

1 tsp chopped thyme

1 tsp chopped rosemary

1 tbsp lemon zest

½ tsp garlic powder

¼ tsp ground nutmeg

Sea salt and freshly ground black pepper, to taste

1 tsp butter

4oz (113g) baby spinach leaves (about 5 cups)

Lemon wedges, for serving

1 Preheat the oven to 425° (220°C). Line a small baking sheet with foil and lightly grease the foil.

2 If the salmon already has the skin removed, then proceed to step 3. To remove the skin, place the salmon on a cutting board. Using a thin, long-bladed knife, at one corner of the salmon and as close to the skin as possible, start to cut between the skin and salmon, keeping the knife blade parallel to the cutting board. When you have enough of the skin to hold onto, place some salt on your fingers to help grasp the salmon skin. Run the knife back and forth until the skin is removed. Discard the skin.

3 Cut the salmon in half (if it's one piece) and tuck the thin section underneath the salmon so it's an even thickness throughout. Place each piece on the baking sheet.

4 In a small bowl, whisk the egg white until lightly frothy. Add the breadcrumbs, Parmesan, parsley, thyme, rosemary, zest, garlic powder, nutmeg, salt, and pepper. Stir until combined. Lightly press the mixture onto the salmon fillets using a fork or your fingers. Bake for 15 minutes, depending on the thickness of the salmon, or until the salmon flakes easily with a fork and is cooked as desired.

5 During the last 2 minutes of the cooking time, prepare the spinach. In a large skillet, melt the butter over medium-high heat. Add the spinach and cook, turning and stirring the spinach, for 1 to 2 minutes or until the spinach is just wilted. Place the spinach on two serving plates, top with the salmon, and serve immediately with lemon wedges.

NUTRITION PER SERVING

CALORIES: **432**   FAT: **23g**   CARBOHYDRATES: **15g**   FIBER: **7g**   SUGARS: **2g**   PROTEIN: **32g**

To make the breadcrumbs, tear a Sesame Seed Bun into pieces, place in a food processor, and process until fine crumbs form. Freeze the leftover crumbs for up to 3 months.

GF DF EF

This souplike coconut milk curry has spiralized zucchini instead of rice noodles. Adjust the curry paste according to your heat tolerance, but note that the flavor for this aromatic curry comes from the curry paste.

RED CHICKEN CURRY WITH ZUCCHINI NOODLES

✕ SERVES: **2**   🕐 PREP: **20 MINUTES**   🔥 COOK: **15 MINUTES**

2 small zucchini (about 10oz/284g total)

2-3 tbsp red curry paste (such as Mae Ploy)

1 cup (250ml) full-fat coconut milk

1 cup chicken broth

2 tbsp coconut aminos

6oz (170g) boneless skinless chicken thighs, chopped

1 tsp avocado oil

2 tbsp fresh lime juice

⅓ cup whole cilantro or Thai basil leaves, plus extra leaves for garnish

⅓ cup bean sprouts or pea shoots

Thinly sliced scallions (optional), for garnish

Lime wedges, for serving

1 Trim the ends from the zucchini and discard. Use a spiralizer or a peeler to create strands of zucchini that resemble noodles. (This makes about 4 cups.) Set aside.

2 In a large sauté pan or wok, combine the curry paste (to taste), coconut milk, broth, and coconut aminos. Bring to a boil, partially covered, then reduce the heat to medium. Add the chicken and cook, uncovered, for 10 minutes or until the chicken is tender and cooked.

3 While the chicken is cooking, in a separate large skillet, heat the oil over medium heat. Add the zucchini noodles. Cook, gently stirring, for 2 minutes or until the noodles are warm.

4 Add the lime juice and cilantro to the noodles. Stir until combined. Place the noodles into warm bowls. Ladle the curry over the noodles.

5 Garnish with extra cilantro, bean sprouts, scallions (if using), and lime wedges. Serve immediately.

Red curry paste is available in the Asian aisle of most grocery stores, at Asian markets, and online.

NUTRITION PER SERVING

CALORIES: **424**   FAT: **32g**   CARBOHYDRATES: **15g**   FIBER: **3g**   SUGARS: **6g**   PROTEIN: **22g**

This soup tastes best with a mixture of mushroom varieties, such as cremini, shiitake, rehydrated wild mushrooms, or small white mushrooms. Serve with Garlic Rolls (page 207) for dipping.

CREAMY MUSHROOM SOUP

SERVES: 4   **PREP: 15 MINUTES**   **COOK: 23 MINUTES**

1 tbsp butter

1 tbsp avocado oil

2lb (907g) mixed mushrooms, sliced (about 10 cups)

1 cup sliced scallions, plus extra for garnish

4 garlic cloves, minced

½ cup dry sherry or dry white wine

1 tsp sea salt

1 tsp freshly ground black pepper

Pinch of ground nutmeg

5 cups chicken or vegetable broth

¾ cup heavy cream

½ tsp xanthan gum

Sour cream (optional), for serving

2 Garlic Rolls (page 207), for serving

1 In a heavy-bottomed stock pot or Dutch oven, melt the butter and oil over medium-high heat. Add the mushrooms, scallions, and garlic. Cook, uncovered, stirring occasionally, for 5 to 7 minutes or until the mushrooms are softened.

2 Add the sherry, salt, pepper, and nutmeg. Cook, stirring, for 1 minute to cook the alcohol off.

3 Add the broth. Bring to boil, and then reduce the heat to medium-low. Simmer, covered, for 10 minutes. Add the heavy cream and stir. Let cool for 5 minutes.

4 Working in two or three batches, spoon the soup into a blender and blend until very smooth. Return the mixture to the same pot. (Alternatively, use an immersion blender directly in the pot.)

5 Add the xanthan gum. Whisk over medium heat until hot and the soup has thickened. Add more broth if the soup becomes too thick. Serve individual portions immediately with a spoonful of sour cream (if using), and half of a roll each for dipping.

NUTRITION PER SERVING (excluding rolls)

CALORIES: **314**   FAT: **24g**   CARBOHYDRATES: **14g**   FIBER: **3g**   SUGARS: **5g**   PROTEIN: **10g**

AMP UP THE FAT AND PROTEIN:
 DOUBLE THE MEATBALL RECIPE.

GF **EF**

This Mediterranean-inspired dish features a slightly spicy tomato sauce and zucchini "noodles." If you're serving fewer than four people, reserve extra meatballs for the Meatball Herb Salad (page 161), or double the meatballs for use later.

GREEK MEATBALLS WITH CHUNKY TOMATO SAUCE

✗ SERVES: **4**   🕐 PREP: **25 MINUTES**   🔥 COOK: **35 MINUTES**

1lb (450g) ground beef (20% fat)

½ cup thinly sliced scallions

4 garlic cloves, minced

2 tbsp chopped dill

1 tbsp chopped oregano, plus extra for garnish

4oz (113g) crumbled feta cheese, plus extra for garnish

1 tsp finely grated lemon zest (optional)

Sea salt and freshly ground black pepper, to taste

3 medium zucchini (about 24oz/ 680g total), thinly sliced lengthwise

1 tbsp olive oil

Chunky tomato sauce:

1 tsp olive oil

2 garlic cloves, minced

1 cup beef or chicken broth

1 (14oz/396g) can fire-roasted diced tomatoes, undrained

2 tbsp tomato paste

½ tsp crushed red pepper

Sea salt and freshly ground black pepper, to taste

Pinch of stevia or granulated monk fruit sweetener (optional)

1 Prepare the chunky tomato sauce. In a medium skillet, heat the oil over medium heat. Add the garlic and cook for 1 minute, or until fragrant. Add the broth, tomatoes with their juices, tomato paste, crushed red pepper, salt, pepper, and stevia (if using). Bring to a boil and reduce to a simmer. Simmer, uncovered, stirring occasionally, for 8 to 10 minutes or until the sauce is thickened. Keep warm.

2 Preheat the oven to 375°F (190°C). Line a baking sheet with parchment paper or foil. Place a greased wire rack on the baking sheet.

3 In a medium bowl, combine the beef, scallions, garlic, dill, oregano, feta, zest (if using), salt, and pepper. Using slightly wet hands to prevent the mixture from sticking, roll the mixture into 24 (1-tablespoon) balls. Arrange on the wire rack. Bake for 22 to 25 minutes or until browned and cooked.

4 While the meatballs are cooking, toss the zucchini in the oil. Sprinkle with salt and pepper. Cook in batches on a hot grill pan until grill marks appear and the zucchini is softened.

5 Arrange the zucchini on 4 serving plates. Add 6 meatballs per serving, top with sauce, and sprinkle with extra feta and oregano leaves for garnish. Serve immediately. Store any extra meatballs in an airtight container in the refrigerator for up to 5 days or in the freezer for up to 3 months.

NUTRITION PER SERVING (6 meatballs)

CALORIES: **471**   FAT: **33g**   CARBOHYDRATES: **17g**   FIBER: **4g**   SUGARS: **11g**   PROTEIN: **28g**

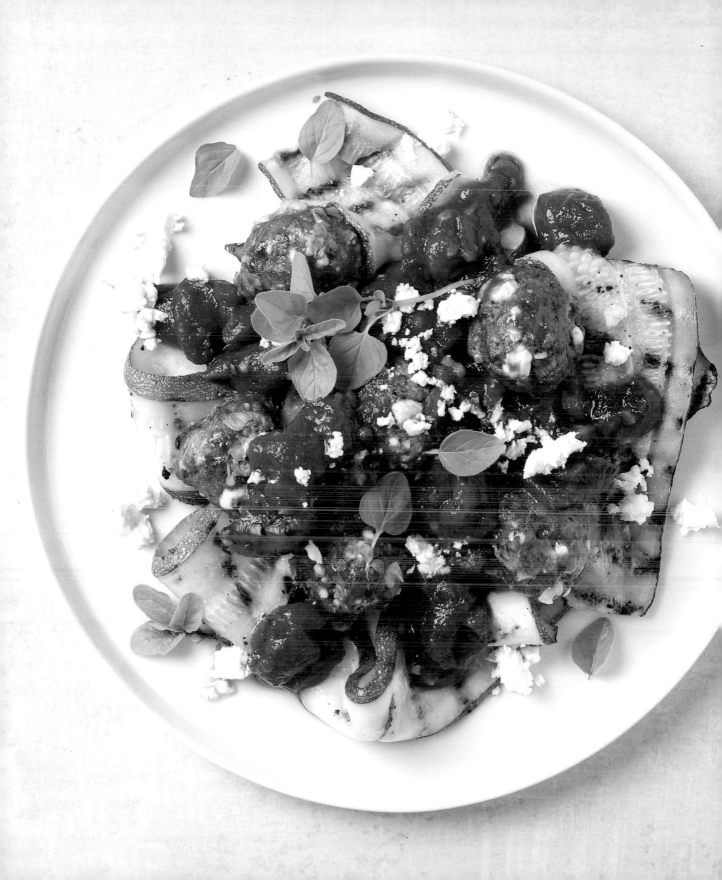

Tender slices of pork with blistered tomatoes are perfectly cooked with asparagus, briny olives, and basil, and then drizzled with balsamic glaze and scattered with Parmesan shavings. Plus, it's all cooked in one pan, making cleanup a cinch!

ONE-PAN MEDITERRANEAN PORK

SERVES: **4**   PREP: **15 MINUTES**   COOK: **20 MINUTES**

1lb (450g) pork shoulder chops (steaks)

2 tsp lemon pepper seasoning

1 tbsp avocado oil

1 tbsp butter

3 garlic cloves, minced

6oz (170g) grape tomatoes, halved

16 pitted Kalamata olives, coarsely chopped

6oz (170g) asparagus, trimmed and cut into 2-in (5cm) pieces

Sea salt and freshly ground black pepper, to taste

¼ cup chopped basil, plus extra leaves for garnish

2 tbsp sugar-free balsamic glaze

½ cup Parmesan cheese shavings

1 Rub the pork all over with the lemon pepper seasoning. Cut into thin slices.

2 In a large skillet over medium-high heat, heat the oil. Cook the pork in two batches for 3 minutes per side until browned. Remove to a plate and cover to keep warm.

3 In the same skillet, melt the butter with the garlic over medium heat. Cook for 1 minute, or until the garlic is fragrant.

4 Add the tomatoes, olives, asparagus, salt, and pepper. Cook, stirring occasionally, for 7 minutes or until the tomatoes are softened and the asparagus is tender-crisp and bright.

5 Add the pork and the chopped basil and stir until combined. Drizzle with the balsamic glaze and sprinkle with Parmesan shavings. Serve immediately.

NUTRITION PER SERVING

CALORIES: **432**   FAT: **31g**   CARBOHYDRATES: **9g**   FIBER: **2g**   SUGARS: **4g**   PROTEIN: **26g**

2 cups refried beans, warmed

Slow-cooked pork:
1½ lb (680g) pork tenderloin
2 tbsp chili powder
2 tbsp smoked paprika
1 tsp sea salt
1 tsp freshly ground black
  pepper, or to taste
½ cup chicken broth
2 tbsp sugar-free barbecue
  sauce, plus extra for serving
1 tbsp Worcestershire sauce

Crunchy slaw:
6 tbsp coconut aminos
¼ cup olive oil
3 tbsp stevia or granulated monk
  fruit sweetener
3 cups shredded red cabbage
3 cups shredded napa cabbage
1 cup thinly sliced scallions
¾ cup chopped cilantro,
  plus extra sprigs for garnish

Creamy sauce:
¼ cup mayonnaise
2 tbsp fresh lime juice
1 tbsp sriracha sauce
2 tsp coconut aminos
2 tsp stevia or granulated monk
  fruit sweetener

Low-carb tortillas:
1¼ cups blanched almond flour
6 tbsp whole psyllium husks
1 tsp baking powder
1 tsp sea salt
4 large egg whites, lightly beaten
½ cup boiling water
2½ tbsp avocado oil, divided

Although the ingredients list may look a little lofty, don't let that dissuade you from making these delicious tacos with homemade tortillas. A tortilla press will give you perfectly round tortillas and makes prep much faster, but you can use a skillet as well. Each section can be made or prepared ahead of time for quick assembly.

SLOW-COOKED PORK AND SLAW TACOS

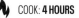

✖ SERVES: **8**   🕐 PREP: **40 MINUTES**   🔥 COOK: **4 HOURS**

1 Prepare the pork. Place the pork on parchment paper for easy cleanup. Rub the pork with the chili powder, paprika, salt, and pepper. In a slow cooker, whisk together the broth, barbecue sauce, and Worcestershire sauce. Place the pork in the slow cooker, and turn to coat. Cover and cook for 4 hours on high, or for 6 to 8 hours on low until the pork is very tender and can be pulled apart. Remove the pork and reserve 3 tablespoons of the broth mixture in the slow cooker, discarding the rest. Shred the pork and return to the slow cooker. Add extra barbecue sauce (if desired). Cover and keep warm.

2 Make the slaw. In a medium bowl, whisk together the coconut aminos, oil, and stevia. Add the red and napa cabbages, scallions, and cilantro, and toss. Cover and refrigerate. Prepare the creamy sauce. In a small bowl, whisk together all of the ingredients until combined. Cover and refrigerate.

3 Make the tortillas. In a medium bowl, mix together almond flour, psyllium, baking powder, and salt. Add the egg whites and mix until well combined. Add the boiling water a little at a time, stirring constantly, to form a soft dough. Cover and let stand for 10 minutes. Roll the dough into 8 equal-size balls. Place one ball between two pieces of parchment paper, dusting the bottom parchment paper with almond flour to prevent sticking. Roll into a 6-inch (15cm) circle. In a small skillet (about 8in/20cm), heat 1 teaspoon avocado oil over medium heat. Carefully add the tortilla, taking care not to tear it. Cook for 30 to 60 seconds on each side until golden brown. Transfer to a plate, and cover to keep warm. Repeat with the remaining dough and avocado oil.

4 Assemble the tacos with refried beans, pulled pork, slaw, and the creamy sauce. Serve immediately with any extra slaw on the side.

NUTRITION PER SERVING (1 taco and ⅛ of the slaw)

CALORIES: **464**   FAT: **29g**   CARBOHYDRATES: **26g**   FIBER: **12g**   SUGARS: **54g**   PROTEIN: **27g**

Sun-dried tomatoes, garlic, fresh basil, mustard, and a hint of chili add flavor to this creamy sauce, which makes the perfect accompaniment to the tender slices of beef.

ONE-PAN CREAMY TUSCAN BEEF

SERVES: 3   **PREP: 15 MINUTES**   **COOK: 15 MINUTES**

1 tbsp avocado oil

12oz (336g) sliced rib eye beef steak (or boneless skinless chicken thighs, thinly sliced)

Sea salt and freshly ground black pepper, to taste

2 garlic cloves, minced

1 cup beef broth

¾ cup heavy whipping cream

2 tsp Dijon mustard

½–1 tsp crushed red pepper

¼ tsp ground nutmeg

½ cup sun-dried tomatoes, drained and cut into strips

¼ cup chopped basil, plus extra leaves for garnish

4oz (113g) baby spinach leaves (about 5 cups)

1 In a large skillet, heat the oil over medium-high heat. Add the beef, salt, and pepper. Cook, stirring occasionally, for 2 to 3 minutes or until the beef is brown. Remove to a bowl using a slotted spoon.

2 Add the garlic and cook for 30 seconds until fragrant. Add the broth, cream, mustard, red pepper flakes (to taste), nutmeg, and sun-dried tomatoes. Cook, stirring occasionally, for 3 to 5 minutes or until the sauce is thickened.

3 Add the basil and stir to combine. Add the spinach and return the beef to the skillet. Stir until the spinach is just wilted. Garnish with basil leaves and serve immediately.

NUTRITION PER SERVING

CALORIES: **528**   FAT: **46g**   CARBOHYDRATES: **8g**   FIBER: **2g**   SUGARS: **1g**   PROTEIN: **25g**

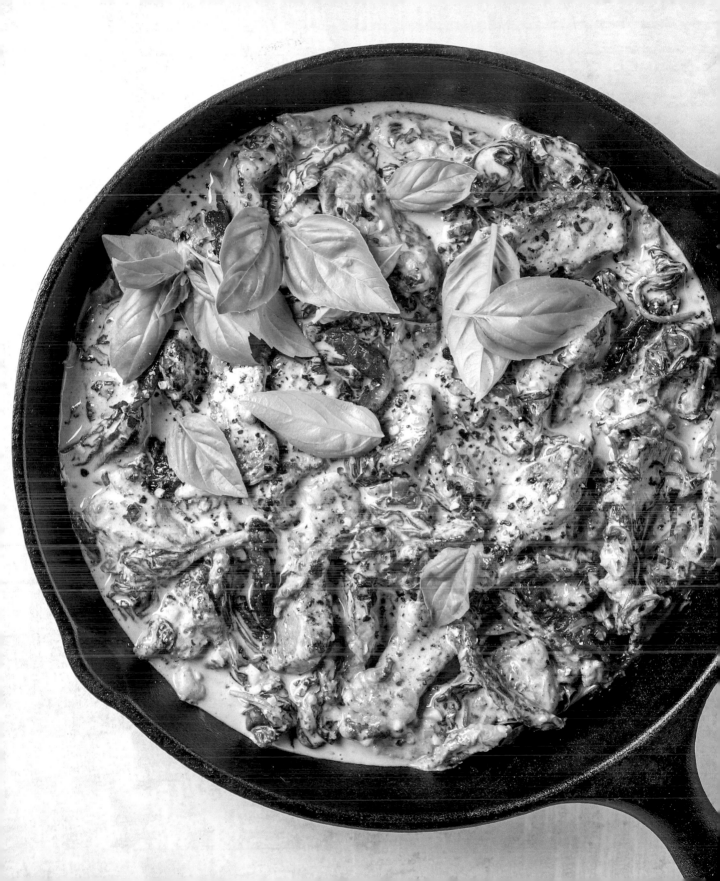

11

SIDES + BASICS

Green beans make a quick and easy side for grilled or roasted meats, taking only minutes to cook. Asparagus can be substituted for the beans.

ALMOND THYME GREEN BEANS

🍴 SERVES: **4**   🕐 PREP: **10 MINUTES**   🔥 COOK: **6 MINUTES**

1lb (450g) green beans, stem ends removed

1 tbsp butter

1 garlic clove, minced

1 tsp chopped thyme, plus extra for garnish

2 tbsp sliced almonds, toasted

Pinch of crushed red pepper

Sea salt, to taste

1 In a large saucepan, boil or steam the beans for 3 to 4 minutes or until bright green and tender-crisp. Drain the green beans in a colander and set aside.

2 Melt the butter in the same saucepan. Add the garlic and cook for 30 seconds or until fragrant.

3 Add the green beans, thyme, almonds, crushed red pepper, and salt. Stir until combined. Arrange on a serving platter. Garnish with extra thyme and serve immediately.

NUTRITION PER SERVING

CALORIES: **59**   FAT: **4g**   CARBOHYDRATES: **6g**   FIBER: **2g**   SUGARS: **3g**   PROTEIN: **2g**

Smooth and comforting—you will not miss the mashed potato in this creamy, cheesy side dish! This is perfect served with grilled or roasted meats, especially the Roasted Herb Chicken and Gravy (page 178).

CHEESY MASHED CAULIFLOWER

✖ MAKES: **ABOUT 3 CUPS**   🕐 PREP: **10 MINUTES**   🔥 COOK: **12 MINUTES**

1 cauliflower head (about 28oz/800g whole), trimmed and cut into florets

1½ cups vegetable or chicken broth

½ cup (0.5oz/14g) finely grated fresh Parmesan cheese, plus extra for garnish

2 tbsp butter, plus extra for serving

2 tbsp sour cream

Pinch of ground nutmeg, plus extra for garnish

Sea salt and white pepper, to taste

1 In a large saucepan, add the cauliflower and broth. Cover and bring to a boil. Reduce the heat to medium. Cook, covered, for 12 minutes, stirring once during the cook time, until the cauliflower is tender. Drain.

2 In the bowl of a food processor, process the cauliflower, Parmesan, butter, sour cream, nutmeg, salt, and pepper until very smooth. (Alternatively, use an immersion blender directly in the pan.)

3 Scrape into a serving bowl. Add a spoonful of butter to the top, if desired. Sprinkle with extra Parmesan and nutmeg, and serve immediately.

NUTRITION PER ⅓ CUP

CALORIES: **98**   FAT: **7g**   CARBOHYDRATES: **5g**   FIBER: **2g**   SUGARS: **2g**   PROTEIN: **5g**

AMP UP THE FAT AND PROTEIN:
 ADD MORE BUTTER
AND BACON.

GF   EF

These sprouts are perfectly crispy and savory, ideal as a side to roasted or grilled proteins. Fresh thyme can be substituted for the rosemary and whole-grain mustard for the Dijon.

MUSTARD ROSEMARY BRUSSELS SPROUTS

SERVES: 4   **PREP: 10 MINUTES**   **COOK: 20 MINUTES**

1lb (450g) Brussels sprouts, trimmed and halved

1 tbsp avocado oil

1 tbsp melted butter

½ tsp garlic power

1 tbsp Dijon mustard

1 tsp stevia or granulated monk fruit sweetener (optional)

½ tsp chopped rosemary

½ tsp sea salt

2 slices cooked bacon, diced

1 Preheat the oven to 400°F (200°C). Line a baking sheet with parchment paper.

2 In a large bowl, toss together the Brussels sprouts, oil, butter, garlic powder, mustard, stevia (if using), rosemary, salt, and bacon. Arrange on the baking sheet in a single layer with the Brussels sprouts cut-side down. Roast for 15 to 20 minutes or until cooked and tender-crisp. Serve immediately.

NUTRITION PER SERVING

CALORIES: **153**   FAT: **11g**   CARBOHYDRATES: **10g**   FIBER: **4g**   SUGARS: **3g**   PROTEIN: **5g**

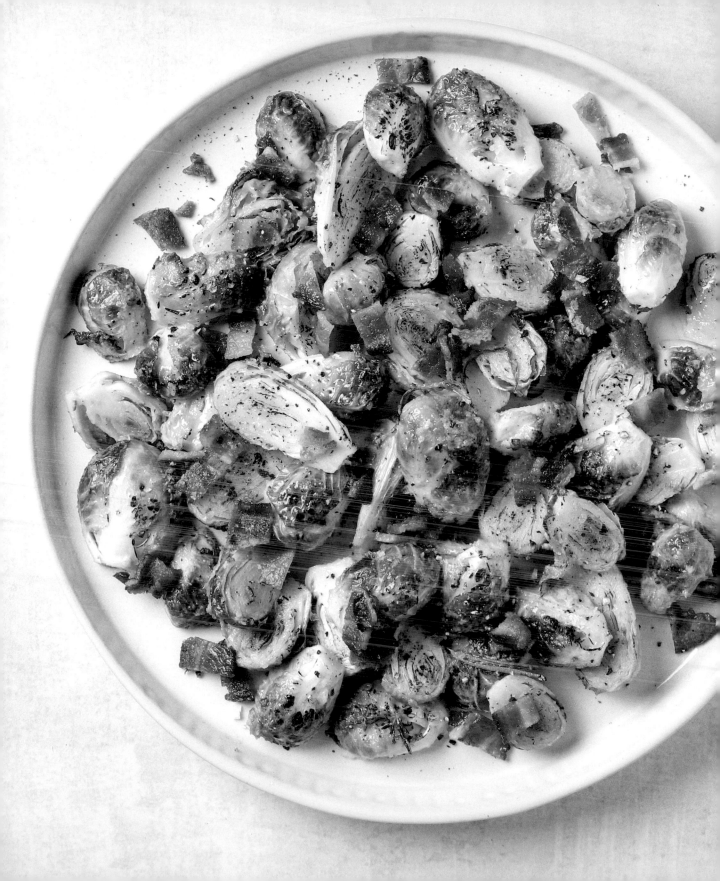

Flavored with onion, garlic, chili powder, and cilantro, this rice is the perfect accompaniment to grilled, roasted, or pan-fried meats.

SPANISH CAULIFLOWER RICE

MAKES: **5 CUPS**   PREP: **15 MINUTES**   COOK: **12 MINUTES**

1 cauliflower head (about 28oz/800g whole), trimmed and cut into florets

1 tbsp butter

1 cup diced red onion

1 jalapeño (optional), diced

2 garlic cloves, minced

2 tsp chili powder

2 tbsp tomato paste

1 cup vegetable or chicken broth

¼ cup coarsely chopped cilantro

Sea salt, to taste

Lime wedges (optional), for serving

1 In the bowl of a food processor, process the cauliflower until finely chopped (but not puréed).

2 In a large skillet, melt the butter over medium heat. Add the onion, jalapeño (if using), and garlic. Cook, stirring occasionally, for 5 minutes or until softened.

3 Add the chili powder and stir for 20 seconds, or until fragrant. Add the tomato paste and broth. Stir until combined.

4 Add the cauliflower rice and stir to combine. Reduce the heat to medium-low. Cover and cook for 5 minutes, stirring once during cooking, until the cauliflower is softened and all the liquid is absorbed.

5 Stir in the cilantro and salt. Serve immediately with lime wedges (if using).

NUTRITION PER ½ CUP

CALORIES: **37**   FAT: **1g**   CARBOHYDRATES: **6g**   FIBER: **2g**   SUGARS: **2g**   PROTEIN: **2g**

Yes, you can still eat bread on a low-carb diet with this unique flour blend! After the bread is cooled, it can be sliced, wrapped, and frozen to have on hand for making toast or sandwiches.

LOW-CARB BREAD LOAF

MAKES: **1 (9 x 5in/ 23 x 13cm) loaf**   PREP: **10 MINUTES**   COOK: **1 HOUR**

12 eggs

½ cup avocado or light olive oil

2 tbsp apple cider vinegar

1¼ cups blanched almond flour

½ cup coconut flour

6 tbsp whole psyllium husks

1 tbsp baking powder

½ tsp sea salt

1 Preheat the oven to 300°F (150°C). Grease and line an 9 x 5 x 3-inch (23 x 13 x 8cm) loaf pan with parchment paper, bringing the paper up over the long sides of the pan to make it easy to remove the cooked loaf.

2 In a medium bowl, whisk the eggs until combined. Add the oil and vinegar. Stir until well combined.

3 In a large bowl, whisk together the almond flour, coconut flour, psyllium, baking powder, and salt.

4 Add the egg mixture to the flour mixture and stir until well combined. Scrape the mixture into the prepared pan. Bake for 1 hour, or until a skewer inserted into the center of the loaf comes out clean. Let stand in the pan for 10 minutes before turning out onto a wire rack to cool. Cool completely before slicing. Cut into 18 (½-in/1.25cm) slices. Store the slices in foil or plastic wrap in the refrigerator for up to 5 days or in the freezer for up to 2 months.

NUTRITION PER SLICE

CALORIES: **167**   FAT: **13g**   CARBOHYDRATES: **7g**   FIBER: **4g**   SUGARS: **1g**   PROTEIN: **6g**

Any leftover buns can be frozen and thawed at room temperature. You can also shape this dough into small, long rolls, like a mini baguette—perfect for Garlic Rolls!

SESAME SEED BUNS

✕ MAKES: **8 ROLLS**   🕐 PREP: **10 MINUTES**   🔥 COOK: **50 MINUTES**

3 cups blanched almond flour

½ cup whole psyllium husks

1 tbsp coconut flour

2 tsp baking soda

1 tsp baking powder

1 tsp stevia or granulated monk fruit sweetener

½ tsp sea salt

1½ cups boiling water

3 tbsp apple cider vinegar

6 large egg whites, lightly beaten

1 egg yolk, lightly beaten

1 tsp sesame seeds

1 Preheat the oven to 375°F (190°C). Line a baking sheet with parchment paper.

2 In a large bowl, combine the almond flour, psyllium, coconut flour, baking soda, baking powder, stevia, and salt. Whisk until thoroughly combined.

3 In a heatproof measuring cup, combine the boiling water and vinegar. Add to the almond flour mixture with the egg whites, and stir to combine. (The mixture will foam.) Continue to stir the mixture until a soft dough forms. Cover and let stand for 2 minutes or until the dough is cool enough to handle.

4 Divide the dough into 8 equal pieces, about 4oz (110g) each. Roll each piece into a ball. Place on the prepared baking sheet. Using your hand, slightly flatten the tops of each ball.

5 Brush the tops with the egg yolk and sprinkle with sesame seeds. Bake for 50 minutes or until browned and the buns sound hollow when tapped. Place on a wire rack to cool. Cool completely before slicing. Store in an airtight container in the refrigerator for up to 5 days or in a freezer bag in the freezer for up to 2 months.

NUTRITION PER SESAME SEED BUN

CALORIES: **312**   FAT: **21g**   CARBOHYDRATES: **23g**   FIBER: **16g**   SUGARS: **2g**   PROTEIN: **12g**

NUTRITION PER GARLIC ROLL

CALORIES: **351**   FAT: **25g**   CARBOHYDRATES: **23g**   FIBER: **16g**   SUGARS: **2g**   PROTEIN: **12g**

Garlic Rolls: On step 4, shape the dough into round buns or small baguettes. Bake according to the recipe directions, brushing the tops of the buns with the egg yolk. Omit the sesame seeds.

When the buns are cooled, preheat the broiler to high and line a baking sheet with foil. Cut the rolls in half and spread the cut sides with a mixture of 3 tablespoons softened butter, 2 minced garlic cloves, and finely chopped fresh herbs, if desired.

Place on a baking sheet and broil 6 inches (15.25cm) under the heat source for 2 minutes or until golden. Serve hot.

3lb (1.3kg) bone-in skin-on chicken drumsticks and thighs

2 large yellow onions, coarsely chopped

4 large carrots, skin on, chopped

4 celery stalks, chopped

3 bay leaves

1 tbsp whole black peppercorns

2 tbsp sea salt

16 cups water

CHICKEN BROTH

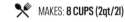

MAKES: 12 CUPS (3qt/3l)   **PREP: 10 MINUTES**   **COOK: 3-24 HOURS**

1 In a large pot, combine the chicken, onions, carrots, celery, bay leaves, peppercorns, and salt. Add the water. Partially cover the pot and bring to a boil over high heat. Reduce the heat to medium-low. Simmer, uncovered, for 3 hours for a lighter broth and up to 24 hours for a richer bone broth.

2 Cool the broth slightly before straining it through a fine-mesh sieve into a large heatproof bowl. Discard the solids. Cover the broth with plastic wrap and refrigerate for 8 hours or overnight.

3 Scrape any solidified fat from the top of the broth and discard. Store in an airtight container in the refrigerator for up to 5 days. Freeze in preportioned and labeled airtight containers for up to 3 months.

NUTRITION PER 1 CUP

CALORIES: **12**   FAT: **1g**   CARBOHYDRATES: **1g**   FIBER: **0g**   SUGARS: **0g**   PROTEIN: **1g**

4 medium carrots, skin on, chopped

2 large yellow onions, chopped

4 celery stalks, chopped

4 garlic cloves, chopped

2 cups sliced mushrooms (5.5oz/155g)

2 bay leaves

3 thyme sprigs

1 tbsp whole black peppercorns

2 cups dry white wine or water

10 cups water

Sea salt, to taste

VEGETABLE BROTH

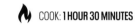

MAKES: 8 CUPS (2qt/2l)   **PREP: 10 MINUTES**   **COOK: 1 HOUR 30 MINUTES**

1 In a large pot or Dutch oven, stir together all of the ingredients. Bring to a boil, and then reduce the heat to medium-low.

2 Simmer, uncovered, for 1 hour 30 minutes.

3 Cool the broth slightly, and then strain through a fine-mesh sieve into a large bowl. Discard the solids. Store in an airtight container in the refrigerator for up to 5 days. Freeze in preportioned and labeled airtight containers for up to 3 months.

NUTRITION PER 1 CUP

CALORIES: **12**   FAT: **0g**   CARBOHYDRATES: **3g**   FIBER: **0g**   SUGARS: **2g**   PROTEIN: **0g**

AMP UP THE FAT AND PROTEIN:
ADD DICED COOKED CHICKEN TO MAKE A QUICK CHICKEN SALAD.

GF **DF** **V**

3 large egg yolks

1½ tbsp fresh lemon juice

1½ tbsp white wine vinegar

½ tsp stevia or granulated monk fruit sweetener (optional)

Sea salt, to taste

1½ cups avocado oil

HOMEMADE MAYONNAISE

 MAKES: **ABOUT 1 ⅔ CUPS**   PREP: **10 MINUTES**   COOK: **NONE**

1 In the bowl of a food processor, process the egg yolks, lemon juice, vinegar, stevia (if using), and salt until combined.

2 With the food processor's motor running, add the oil in a slow, steady stream down the feed shoot until the mixture is thick and pale. (This step should take about 4 minutes; you must add the oil very slowly, or it will not emulsify.) Spoon the mayonnaise into clean jars, seal, and store in the refrigerator for up to 2 weeks.

NUTRITION PER 1 TABLESPOON

CALORIES: **18**   FAT: **2g**   CARBOHYDRATES: **1g**   FIBER: **0g**   SUGARS: **1g**   PROTEIN: **1g**

AMP UP THE FAT AND PROTEIN:
ADJUST THE BUTTER, CREAM, AND MCT OIL TO YOUR LIKING.

GF **EF** **V**

1 cup hot brewed coffee

1 tbsp unsalted butter (optional)

1 tbsp heavy whipping cream

1 tsp MCT oil

KETO COFFEE

SERVES: **1**   PREP: **3 MINUTES**   COOK: **NONE**

In a large coffee cup, stir together all of the ingredients. For a frothier drink like a latte, blend for 20 to 30 seconds. Drink hot.

If you have a more sensitive stomach, replace some of the MCT oil with additional cream.

NUTRITION PER SERVING (including butter)

CALORIES: **196**   FAT: **22g**   CARBOHYDRATES: **0g**   FIBER: **0g**   SUGARS: **0g**   PROTEIN: **1g**

NUTRITION PER SERVING (excluding butter)

CALORIES: **95**   FAT: **10g**   CARBOHYDRATES: **0g**   FIBER: **0g**   SUGARS: **0g**   PROTEIN: **1g**

ENDNOTES

Introduction

1. Gill, Shubhroz, and Satchidananda Panda. "A Smartphone App Reveals Erratic Diurnal Eating Patterns in Humans That Can Be Modulated for Health Benefits." *Cell Metabolism* 22, no. 5 (November 3, 2015): 789–98. https://doi.org/10.1016/j.cmet.2015.09.005.

2. Panda, Satchidananda. "Circadian Physiology of Metabolism." *Science* 354, no. 6315 (November 25, 2016): 1008–15. https://doi.org/10.1126/science.aah4967.

Chapter 1

1. Harnack, Lisa, Lyn Steffen, Donna K. Arnett, Shujun Gao, and Russell V. Luepker. "Accuracy of Estimation of Large Food Portions." *Journal of the American Dietetic Association* 104, no. 5 (May 2004): 804–06. https://doi.org/10.1016/j.jada.2004.02.026.

2. Cook, Adrian, Jane Pryer, and Prakash Shetty. "The Problem of Accuracy in Dietary Surveys. Analysis of the over 65 UK National Diet and Nutrition Survey." *Journal of Epidemiology & Community Health* 54, no. 8 (August 1, 2000): 611–16. https://doi.org/10.1136/jech.54.8.611.

3. "Diet History Questionnaire III (DHQ III)." Epidemiology and Genomic Research Program. NIH National Cancer Institute: Division of Cancer Control & Population Sciences, last modified March 20, 2020. https://epi.grants.cancer.gov/dhq3/.

4. Gill, Shubhroz, and Satchidananda Panda. "A Smartphone App Reveals Erratic Diurnal Eating Patterns in Humans That Can Be Modulated for Health Benefits." *Cell Metabolism* 22, no. 5 (November 3, 2015): 789–98. https://doi.org/10.1016/j.cmet.2015.09.005.

5. Sanger, Gareth J., Per M. Hellström, and Erik Näslund. "The Hungry Stomach: Physiology, Disease, and Drug Development Opportunities." *Frontiers in Pharmacology* 1, no. 145 (February 18, 2011). https://doi.org/10.3389/fphar.2010.00145.

6. Longo, Valter D., and Satchidananda Panda. "Fasting, Circadian Rhythms, and Time-Restricted Feeding in Healthy Lifespan." *Cell Metabolism* 23, no. 6 (June 14, 2016): 1048–59. https://doi.org/10.1016/j.cmet.2016.06.001.

7. Bush, Bradley, and Tori Hudson. "The Role of Cortisol in Sleep: The Hypothalamic-Pituitary-Adrenal (HPA) Axis Interacts with Sleep in Multiple Ways. This Article Reviews the Effects of the HPA Axis on Sleep and the Converse." *Natural Medicine Journal* 2, no. 6 (June 2010).

8. Astbury, Nerys M., Moira A. Taylor, and Ian A. Macdonald. "Breakfast Consumption Affects Appetite, Energy Intake, and the Metabolic and Endocrine Responses to Foods Consumed Later in the Day in Male Habitual Breakfast Eaters." *The Journal of Nutrition* 141, no. 7 (July 2011): 1381–89. https://doi.org/10.3945/jn.110.128645.

9. Levitsky, David A., and Carly R. Pacanowski. "Effect of Skipping Breakfast on Subsequent Energy Intake." *Physiology & Behavior* 119 (July 2, 2013): 9–16. https://doi.org/10.1016/j.physbeh.2013.05.006.

10. Dawson, John, Amy Alcorn, Michelle Cardel, Arne Astrup, Marie-Claude St-Onge, Emily J. Dhurandhar, Lesli H. Larsen, et al. "The Effectiveness of Breakfast Recommendations on Weight Loss: a Randomized Controlled Trial." *The American Journal of Clinical Nutrition* 100, no. 2 (August 2014): 507–13. https://doi.org/10.3945/ajcn.114.089573.

Chapter 2

1. Bier, Dennis M., Doris Derelian, J. Bruce German, David L. Katz, Russell R. Pate, and Kimberly M. Thompson. "Improving Compliance With Dietary Recommendations." *Nutrition Today* 43, no. 5 (2008): 180–87. https://doi.org/10.1097/01.nt.0000338564.14317.69.

2. Gill, Shubhroz, and Satchidananda Panda. "A Smartphone App Reveals Erratic Diurnal Eating Patterns in Humans That Can Be Modulated for Health Benefits." *Cell Metabolism* 22, no. 5 (November 3, 2015): 789–98. https://doi.org/10.1016/j.cmet.2015.09.005.

3. Barnosky, Adrienne R., Kristin K. Hoddy, Terry G. Unterman, and Krista A. Varady. "Intermittent Fasting vs Daily Calorie Restriction for Type 2 Diabetes Prevention: a Review of Human Findings." *Translational Research* 164, no. 4 (October 2014): 302–11. https://doi.org/10.1016/j.trsl.2014.05.013.

4. Lammers, Laureen A., Roos Achterbergh, Johannes A. Romijn, and Ron A. A. Mathôt. "The Effects of Fasting on Drug Metabolism." *Expert Opinion on Drug Metabolism & Toxicology* 16, no. 1 (2020): 79–85. https://doi.org/10.1080/17425255.2020.1706728.

5. Kumar, Sushil, and Gurcharan Kaur. "Intermittent Fasting Dietary Restriction Regimen Negatively Influences Reproduction in Young Rats: A Study of Hypothalamo-Hypophysial-Gonadal Axis." *PLoS ONE* 8, no. 1 (2013). https://doi.org/10.1371/journal.pone.0052416.

6. Meczekalski, B., K. Katulski, A. Czyzyk, A. Podfigurna-Stopa, and M. Maciejewska-Jeske. "Functional Hypothalamic Amenorrhea and Its Influence on Women's Health." *Journal of Endocrinological Investigation* 37, no. 11 (2014): 1049–56. https://doi.org/10.1007/s40618-014-0169-3

7. Ikhsan, Muhammad. "The Relationship Between Ramadan Fasting with Menstrual Cycle Pattern Changes in Teenagers." *Middle East Fertility Society Journal* 22, no. 1 (March 2017): 43–47. https://doi.org/10.18502/kme.v1i1.545.

8. Nair, Pradeep M. K., and Pranav G. Khawale. "Role of Therapeutic Fasting in Women's Health: An Overview." *Journal of Mid-life Health* 7, no. 2 (April 2016): 61–64. https://doi.org/10.4103/0976-7800.185325.

9. Dubois, Lise, Manon Girard, Monique Potvin Kent, Anna Farmer, and Fabiola Tatone-Tokuda. "Breakfast Skipping Is Associated with Differences in Meal Patterns,

Macronutrient Intakes and Overweight among Pre-School Children." *Public Health Nutrition* 12, no. 1 (January 2009): 19–28. https://doi.org/10.1017/s1368980008001894.

10. Giovannini, Marcello, Carlo Agostoni, and Raanan Shamir. "Symposium Overview: Do We All Eat Breakfast and Is It Important?" *Critical Reviews in Food Science and Nutrition* 50, no. 2 (February 2010): 97–99. https://doi.org/10.1080/10408390903467373.

Chapter 3

1. "Adult Obesity Facts." Centers for Disease Control and Prevention, last modified February 27, 2020. https://www.cdc.gov/obesity/data/adult.html.

2. Gould, Skye. "6 Charts That Show How Much More Americans Eat than They Used To." Business Insider, last modified May 10, 2017. https://www.businessinsider.com/daily-calories-americans-eat-increase-2016-07.

3. Varady, K. A. "Intermittent versus Daily Calorie Restriction: Which Diet Regimen Is More Effective for Weight Loss?" *Obesity Reviews* 12, no. 7 (March 17, 2011): e593–e601. https://doi.org/10.1111/j.1467-789x.2011.00873.x.

4. Gardner, Christopher D., John F. Trepanowski, Liana C. Del Gobbo, Michelle E. Hauser, Joseph Rigdon, John P. A. Ioannidis, Manisha Desai, and Abby C. King. "Effect of Low-Fat vs Low-Carbohydrate Diet on 12-Month Weight Loss in Overweight Adults and the Association With Genotype Pattern or Insulin Secretion." *JAMA* 319, no. 7 (February 20, 2018): 667–79. https://doi.org/10.1001/jama.2018.0245.

5. "Insulin Resistance & Prediabetes." National Institute of Diabetes and Digestive and Kidney Diseases. U.S. Department of Health and Human Services, last modified May 2018. https://www.niddk.nih.gov/health-information/diabetes/overview/what-is-diabetes/prediabetes-insulin-resistance.

6. Feinman, Richard D., Wendy K. Pogozelski, Arne Astrup, Richard K. Bernstein, Eugene J. Fine, Eric C. Westman, Anthony Accurso, et al. "Dietary Carbohydrate Restriction as the First Approach in Diabetes Management: Critical Review and Evidence Base." *Nutrition. The International Journal of Applied and Basic Nutritional Sciences* 31, no. 1 (January 2015): 1–13. https://doi.org/https://doi.org/10.1016/j.nut.2014.06.011.

7. Sutton, Elizabeth F., Robbie Beyl, Kate S. Early, William T. Cefalu, Eric Ravussin, and Courtney M. Peterson. "Early Time-Restricted Feeding Improves Insulin Sensitivity, Blood Pressure, and Oxidative Stress Even without Weight Loss in Men with Prediabetes." *Cell Metabolism* 27, no. 6 (June 5, 2018): 1212–21. https://doi.org/10.1016/j.cmet.2018.04.010.

8. Wilkinson, Michael J., Emily N.C. Manoogian, Adena Zadourian, Hannah Lo, Savannah Fakhouri, Azarin Shoghi, Xinran Wang, et al. "Ten-Hour Time-Restricted Eating Reduces Weight, Blood Pressure, and Atherogenic Lipids in Patients with Metabolic Syndrome." *Cell Metabolism* 31, no. 1 (January 7, 2020): 92–104. https://doi.org/10.1016/j.cmet.2019.11.004.

9. Horne, Benjamin D., Heidi T. May, Jeffrey L. Anderson, Abdallah G. Kfoury, Beau M. Bailey, Brian S. McClure, Dale G. Renlund, et al. "Usefulness of Routine Periodic Fasting to Lower Risk of Coronary Artery Disease in Patients Undergoing Coronary Angiography." *The American Journal of Cardiology* 102, no. 7 (October 1, 2008): 814–19. https://doi.org/10.1016/j.amjcard.2008.05.021.

10. Cabo, Rafael de, and Mark P. Mattson. "Effects of Intermittent Fasting on Health, Aging, and Disease." *The New England Journal of Medicine* 381, no. 26 (December 26, 2019): 2541–51. https://doi.org/10.1056/NEJMra1905136.

11. Longo, Valter D., and Mark P. Mattson. "Fasting: Molecular Mechanisms and Clinical Applications." *Cell Metabolism* 19, no. 2 (February 4, 2014): 181–92. https://doi.org/10.1016/j.cmet.2013.12.008.

12. Lee, C., L. Raffaghello, S. Brandhorst, F. M. Safdie, G. Bianchi, A. Martin-Montalvo, V. Pistoia, et al. "Fasting Cycles Retard Growth of Tumors and Sensitize a Range of Cancer Cell Types to Chemotherapy." *Science Translational Medicine* 4, no. 124 (March 7, 2012). https://doi.org/10.1126/scitranslmed.3003293.

13. Marinac, Catherine R., Sandahl H. Nelson, Caitlin I. Breen, Sheri J. Hartman, Loki Natarajan, John P. Pierce, Shirley W. Flatt, Dorothy D. Sears, and Ruth E. Patterson. "Prolonged Nightly Fasting and Breast Cancer Prognosis." *JAMA Oncology* 2, no. 8 (August 2016): 1049–55. https://doi.org/10.1001/jamaoncol.2016.0164.

14. Marinac, Catherine R., Dorothy D. Sears, Loki Natarajan, Linda C. Gallo, Caitlin I. Breen, and Ruth E. Patterson. "Frequency and Circadian Timing of Eating May Influence Biomarkers of Inflammation and Insulin Resistance Associated with Breast Cancer Risk." *PLoS ONE* 10, no. 8 (August 25, 2015). https://doi.org/10.1371/journal.pone.0136240.

15. Zauner, Christian, Bruno Schneeweiss, Alexander Kranz, Christian Madl, Klaus Ratheiser, Ludwig Kramer, Erich Roth, Barbara Schneider, and Kurt Lenz. "Resting Energy Expenditure in Short-Term Starvation Is Increased as a Result of an Increase in Serum Norepinephrine." *The American Journal of Clinical Nutrition* 71, no. 6 (June 2000): 1511–15. https://doi.org/10.1093/ajcn/71.6.1511.

16. Ho, K. Y., J. D. Veldhuis, M. L. Johnson, R. Furlanetto, W. S. Evans, K. G. Alberti, and M. O. Thorner. "Fasting Enhances Growth Hormone Secretion and Amplifies the Complex Rhythms of Growth Hormone Secretion in Man." *Journal of Clinical Investigation* 81, no. 4 (April 1988): 968–75. https://doi.org/10.1172/jci113450.

17. Olarescu, Nicoleta Cristina, Kavinga Gunawardane, Troels Krarup Hansen, Niels Møller, and Jens Otto Lunde Jørgensen. "Normal Physiology of Growth Hormone in Adults." Endotext [Internet]. U.S. National Library of Medicine, October 16, 2019. https://www.ncbi.nlm.nih.gov/books/NBK279056/.

18. Schönfeld, Peter, and Georg Reiser. "Why Does Brain Metabolism Not Favor Burning of Fatty Acids to Provide Energy? - Reflections on Disadvantages of the Use of Free Fatty Acids as Fuel for Brain." *Journal of Cerebral Blood Flow & Metabolism* 33, no. 10 (October 2013): 1493–99. https://doi.org/10.1038/jcbfm.2013.128.

19. Singh, Rumani, Dinesh Lakhanpal, Sushil Kumar, Sandeep Sharma, Hardeep Kataria, Manpreet Kaur, and Gurcharan Kaur. "Late-Onset Intermittent Fasting Dietary Restriction as a Potential Intervention to Retard Age-Associated Brain Function Impairments in Male Rats." *Age* 34, no. 4 (August 2012): 917–33. https://doi.org/10.1007/s11357-011-9289-2.

20. Fontan-Lozano, A., J. L. Saez-Cassanelli, M. C. Inda, M. De Los Santos-Arteaga, S. A. Sierra-Dominguez, G. Lopez-Lluch, J. M. Delgado-Garcia, and A. M. Carrion. "Caloric Restriction Increases Learning Consolidation and Facilitates Synaptic Plasticity through Mechanisms Dependent on NR2B Subunits of the NMDA Receptor." *Journal of Neuroscience* 27, no. 38 (September 19, 2007): 10185–95. https://doi.org/10.1523/jneurosci.2757-07.2007.

21. Fond, Guillaume, Alexandra Macgregor, Marion Leboyer, and Andreas Michalsen. "Fasting in Mood Disorders: Neurobiology and Effectiveness. A Review of the Literature." *Psychiatry Research* 209, no. 3 (2013): 253–58. https://doi.org/10.1016/j.psychres.2012.12.018.

22. Kuehn, Bridget M. "In Alzheimer Research, Glucose Metabolism Moves to Center Stage." *JAMA* 323, no. 4 (January 8, 2020): 297–99. https://doi.org/10.1001/jama.2019.20939.

23. "Heart Disease Facts." Centers for Disease Control and Prevention, last modified December 2, 2019. https://www.cdc.gov/heartdisease/facts.htm.

24. Bhutani, Surabhi, Monica C. Klempel, Reed A. Berger, and Krista A. Varady. "Improvements in Coronary Heart Disease Risk Indicators by Alternate-Day Fasting Involve Adipose Tissue Modulations." *Obesity* 18, no. 11 (November 2010): 2152–59. https://doi.org/10.1038/oby.2010.54.

25. Azevedo, Fernanda Reis De, Dimas Ikeoka, and Bruno Caramelli. "Effects of Intermittent Fasting on Metabolism in Men." *Revista da Associação Médica Brasileira (English Edition)* 59, no. 2 (2013): 167–73. https://doi.org/10.1016/s2255-4823(13)70451-x.

26. Varady, Krista A., Surabhi Bhutani, Emily C. Church, and Monica C. Klempel. "Short-Term Modified Alternate-Day Fasting: a Novel Dietary Strategy for Weight Loss and Cardioprotection in Obese Adults." *The American Journal of Clinical Nutrition* 90, no. 5 (November 2009): 1138–43. https://doi.org/10.3945/ajcn.2009.28380.

27. Han, Young-Min, Tatiana Bedarida, Ye Ding, Brian K. Somba, Qiulun Lu, Qilong Wang, Ping Song, and Ming-Hui Zou. "ß-Hydroxybutyrate Prevents Vascular Senescence through HnRNP A1-Mediated Upregulation of Oct4." *Molecular Cell* 71, no. 6 (September 20, 2018): 1064–78. https://doi.org/10.1016/j.molcel.2018.07.036.

28. Trepanowski, John F., and Richard J. Bloomer. "The Impact of Religious Fasting on Human Health." *Nutrition Journal* 9, no. 1 (November 22, 2010). https://doi.org/10.1186/1475-2891-9-57.

29. Alirezaei, Mehrdad, Christopher C. Kemball, Claudia T. Flynn, Malcolm R. Wood, J. Lindsay Whitton, and William B. Kiosses. "Short-Term Fasting Induces Profound Neuronal Autophagy." *Autophagy* 6, no. 6 (August 16, 2010): 702–10. https://doi.org/10.4161/auto.6.6.12376.

30. Jamshed, Humaira, Robbie A. Beyl, Deborah L. Della Manna, Eddy S. Yang, Eric Ravussin, and Courtney M. Peterson. "Early Time-Restricted Feeding Improves 24-Hour Glucose Levels and Affects Markers of the Circadian Clock, Aging, and Autophagy in Humans." *Nutrients* 11, no. 6 (2019): 1234. https://doi.org/10.3390/nu11061234.

31. Quigley, Eamonn M. M. "Gut Bacteria in Health and Disease." *Gastroenterology & Hepatology* 9, no. 9 (September 2013): 560–69.

32. Guinane, Caitriona M., and Paul D. Cotter. "Role of the Gut Microbiota in Health and Chronic Gastrointestinal Disease: Understanding a Hidden Metabolic Organ." *Therapeutic Advances in Gastroenterology* 6, no. 4 (March 26, 2013): 295–308. https://doi.org/10.1177/1756283x13482996.

33. Kaczmarek, Jennifer L., Sharon V. Thompson, and Hannah D. Holscher. "Complex Interactions of Circadian Rhythms, Eating Behaviors, and the Gastrointestinal Microbiota and Their Potential Impact on Health." *Nutrition Reviews* 75, no. 9 (August 7, 2017): 673–82. https://doi.org/10.1093/nutrit/nux036.

34. Patterson, Ruth E., and Dorothy D. Sears. "Metabolic Effects of Intermittent Fasting." *Annual Review of Nutrition* 37, no. 1 (August 2017): 371–93. https://doi.org/10.1146/annurev-nutr-071816-064634.

35. Mu, Qinghui, Jay Kirby, Christopher M. Reilly, and Xin M. Luo. "Leaky Gut As a Danger Signal for Autoimmune Diseases." *Frontiers in Immunology* 8 (May 23, 2017): 598. https://doi.org/10.3389/fimmu.2017.00598.

36. Wolf, George. "Calorie Restriction Increases Life Span: A Molecular Mechanism." *Nutrition Reviews* 64, no. 2 (February 1, 2006): 89–92. https://doi.org/10.1111/j.1753-4887.2006.tb00192.x.

37. Barzilai, N., and A. Bartke. "Biological Approaches to Mechanistically Understand the Healthy Life Span Extension Achieved by Calorie Restriction and Modulation of Hormones." *The Journals of Gerontology Series A: Biological Sciences and Medical Sciences* 64A, no. 2 (February 2009): 187–91. https://doi.org/10.1093/gerona/gln061.

38. Mitchell, Sarah J., Michel Bernier, Julie A. Mattison, Miguel A. Aon, Tamzin A. Kaiser, R. Michael Anson, Yuji Ikeno, Rozalyn M. Anderson, Donald K. Ingram, and Rafael De Cabo. "Daily Fasting Improves Health and Survival in Male Mice Independent of Diet Composition and Calories." *Cell Metabolism* 29, no. 1 (January 8, 2019): 221–28. https://doi.org/10.1016/j.cmet.2018.08.011.

39. Srikanthan, Preethi, and Arun S. Karlamangla. "Muscle Mass Index As a Predictor of Longevity in Older Adults." *The American Journal of Medicine* 127, no. 6 (June 2014): 547–53. https://doi.org/10.1016/j.amjmed.2014.02.007.

40. Tinsley, Grant M., and Paul M. La Bounty. "Effects of Intermittent Fasting on Body Composition and Clinical Health Markers in Humans." *Nutrition Reviews* 73, no. 10 (October 2015): 661–74. https://doi.org/10.1093/nutrit/nuv041.

41. Owen, Oliver E., Philip Felig, Alfred P. Morgan, John Wahren, and George F. Cahill. "Liver and Kidney Metabolism during Prolonged Starvation." *Journal of Clinical Investigation* 48, no. 3 (March 1, 1969): 574–83. https://doi.org/10.1172/jci106016.

42. Benedict, Francis Gano, Harry Winfred Goodall, James Earle Ash, Herbert Sidney Langfeld, Arthur Isaac Kendall, and Harld Leonard Higgins. "Protein Katabolism." In *A Study of Prolonged Fasting,* 400–01. Carnegie Institution of Washington, 1915.

43. Elia, Marinos, Jason Payne-James, George K. Grimble, and David B. A. Silk. "Metabolic Response to Starvation, Injury and Sepsis." Essay. In *Artificial Nutrition Support in Clinical Practice,* 2nd ed. Cambridge: Cambridge University Press, 2012.

Chapter 4

1. Gill, Shubhroz, and Satchidananda Panda. "A Smartphone App Reveals Erratic Diurnal Eating Patterns in Humans That Can Be Modulated for Health Benefits." *Cell Metabolism* 22, no. 5 (November 3, 2015): 789–98. https://doi.org/10.1016/j.cmet.2015.09.005.

2. Patterson, Ruth E., and Dorothy D. Sears. "Metabolic Effects of Intermittent Fasting." *Annual Review of Nutrition* 37, no. 1 (August 2017): 371–93. https://doi.org/10.1146/annurev-nutr-071816-064634.

3. Fothergill, Erin, Juen Guo, Lilian Howard, Jennifer C. Kerns, Nicolas D. Knuth, Robert Brychta, Kong Y. Chen, et al. "Persistent Metabolic Adaptation 6 Years after 'The Biggest Loser' Competition." *Obesity* 24, no. 8 (May 2, 2016): 1612–19. https://doi.org/10.1002/oby.21538.

4. Alhamdan, B. A., A. Garcia-Alvarez, A. H. Alzahrnai, J. Karanxha, D. R. Stretchberry, K. J. Contrera, A. F. Utria, and L. J. Cheskin. "Alternate-Day versus Daily Energy Restriction Diets: Which Is More Effective for Weight Loss? A Systematic Review and Meta Analysis." *Obesity Science & Practice* 2, no. 3 (July 15, 2016): 293–302. https://doi.org/10.1002/osp4.52.

5. Klempel, Monica C., Surabhi Bhutani, Marian Fitzgibbon, Sally Freels, and Krista A. Varady. "Dietary and Physical Activity Adaptations to Alternate Day Modified Fasting: Implications for Optimal Weight Loss." *Nutrition Journal* 9, no. 35 (September 3, 2010). https://doi.org/10.1186/1475-2891-9-35.

6. Stekovic, Slaven, Sebastian J. Hofer, Norbert Tripolt, Miguel A. Aon, Philipp Royer, Lukas Pein, Julia T. Stadler, et al. "Alternate Day Fasting Improves Physiological and Molecular Markers of Aging in Healthy, Non-Obese Humans." *Cell Metabolism* 30, no. 3 (September 3, 2019): 462–76. https://doi.org/10.1016/j.cmet.2020.02.011.

7. Varady, Krista A., Surabhi Bhutani, Emily C. Church, and Monica C. Klempel. "Short-Term Modified Alternate-Day Fasting: a Novel Dietary Strategy for Weight Loss and Cardioprotection in Obese Adults." *The American Journal of Clinical Nutrition* 90, no. 5 (November 2009): 1138–43. https://doi.org/10.3945/ajcn.2009.28380.

8. Elia, Marinos, Jason Payne-James, George K. Grimble, and David B. A. Silk. "Metabolic Response to Starvation, Injury and Sepsis." Essay. In *Artificial Nutrition Support in Clinical Practice,* 2nd ed. Cambridge: Cambridge University Press, 2012.

9. Harvie, M. N., M. Pegington, M. P. Mattson, J. Frystyk, B. Dillon, G. Evans, J. Cuzick, et al. "The Effects of Intermittent or Continuous Energy Restriction on Weight Loss and Metabolic Disease Risk Markers: a Randomized Trial in Young Overweight Women." *International Journal of Obesity* 35, no. 5 (May 2011): 714–27. https://doi.org/10.1038/ijo.2010.171.

10. Sinha, Rohit A., Benjamin L. Farah, Brijesh K. Singh, Monowarul M. Siddique, Ying Li, Yajun Wu, Olga R. Ilkayeva, et al. "Caffeine Stimulates Hepatic Lipid Metabolism by the Autophagy-Lysosomal Pathway in Mice." *Hepatology* 59, no. 4 (April 2014): 1366–80. https://doi.org/10.1002/hep.26667.

11. Pietrocola, Federico, Shoaib Ahmad Malik, Guillermo Mariño, Erika Vacchelli, Laura Senovilla, Kariman Chaba, Mireia Niso-Santano, Maria Chiara Maiuri, Frank Madeo, and Guido Kroemer. "Coffee Induces Autophagy in Vivo." *Cell Cycle* 13, no. 12 (March 2014): 1987–94. https://doi.org/10.4161/cc.28929.

12. Korbonits Márta, David Blaine, Marinos Elia, and Jeremy Powell-Tuck. "Metabolic and Hormonal Changes during the Refeeding Period of Prolonged Fasting." *European Journal of Endocrinology* 157, no. 2 (August 1, 2007): 157–66. https://doi.org/10.1530/eje-06-0740.

Chapter 5

1. Moro, Tatiana, Grant Tinsley, Antonino Bianco, Giuseppe Marcolin, Quirico Francesco Pacelli, Giuseppe Battaglia, Antonio Palma, Paulo Gentil, Marco Neri, and Antonio Paoli. "Effects of Eight Weeks of Time-Restricted Feeding (16/8) on Basal Metabolism, Maximal Strength, Body Composition, Inflammation, and Cardiovascular Risk Factors in Resistance-Trained Males." *Journal of Translational Medicine* 14, no. 1 (2016). https://doi.org/10.1186/s12967-016-1044-0.

2. Tinsley, Grant M., M. Lane Moore, Austin J. Graybeal, Antonio Paoli, Youngdeok Kim, Joaquin U. Gonzales, John R. Harry, Trisha A. Vandusseldorp, Devin N. Kennedy, and Megan R. Cruz. "Time-Restricted Feeding plus Resistance Training in Active Females: a Randomized Trial." *The American Journal of Clinical Nutrition* 110, no. 3 (September 2019): 628–40. https://doi.org/10.1093/ajcn/nqz126.

3. Cantó, Carles, Keir Menzies, and Johan Auwerx. "NAD+ Metabolism and the Control of Energy Homeostasis: A Balancing Act between Mitochondria and the Nucleus." *Cell Metabolism* 22, no. 1 (July 7, 2015): 31–53. https://doi.org/10.1016/j.cmet.2015.05.023.

4. Panda, Satchidananda, and Rhonda Patrick. "Shift Work as a Carcinogen and How Time-Restricted Eating May Help: Satchin Panda." FoundMyFitness, last modified July 12, 2019. https://www.foundmyfitness.com/episodes/shift-work-as-a-carcinogen-and-how-time-restricted-eating-may-help.

5. Anton, Stephen D., Stephanie A. Lee, William T. Donahoo, Christian Mclaren, Todd Manini, Christiaan Leeuwenburgh, and Marco Pahor. "The Effects of Time Restricted Feeding on Overweight, Older Adults: A Pilot Study." *Nutrients* 11, no. 7 (2019): 1500. https://doi.org/10.3390/nu11071500.

6. Sutton, Elizabeth F., Robbie Beyl, Kate S. Early, William T. Cefalu, Eric Ravussin, and Courtney M. Peterson. "Early Time-Restricted Feeding Improves Insulin Sensitivity, Blood Pressure, and Oxidative Stress Even without Weight Loss in Men with Prediabetes." *Cell Metabolism* 27, no. 6 (June 5, 2018): 1212–21. https://doi.org/10.1016/j.cmet.2018.04.010.

Chapter 6

1. "How Much Is Too Much?: The Growing Concern over Too Much Added Sugar in Our Diets." Sugar Science. University of California San Francisco. Accessed July 7, 2020. https://sugarscience.ucsf.edu/the-growing-concern-of-overconsumption.html.

2. Foster-Schubert, Karen E., Joost Overduin, Catherine E. Prudom, Jianhua Liu, Holly S. Callahan, Bruce D. Gaylinn, Michael O. Thorner, and David E. Cummings. "Acyl and Total Ghrelin Are Suppressed Strongly by Ingested Proteins, Weakly by Lipids, and Biphasically by Carbohydrates." *The Journal of Clinical Endocrinology & Metabolism* 93, no. 5 (May 1, 2008): 1971–79. https://doi.org/10.1210/jc.2007-2289.

3. "Adult Obesity Prevalence Maps." Centers for Disease Control and Prevention, last modified October 29, 2019. https://www.cdc.gov/obesity/data/prevalence-maps.html.

4. "Adult Obesity Facts." Centers for Disease Control and Prevention, last modified June 29, 2020. https://www.cdc.gov/obesity/data/adult.html.

5. Hallberg, Sarah J., Amy L. Mckenzie, Paul T. Williams, Nasir H. Bhanpuri, Anne L. Peters, Wayne W. Campbell, Tamara L. Hazbun, et al. "Author Correction: Effectiveness and Safety of a Novel Care Model for the Management of Type 2 Diabetes at 1 Year: An Open-Label, Non-Randomized, Controlled Study." *Diabetes Therapy* 9 (2018): 583–612. https://doi.org/10.1007/s13300-018-0386-4.

6. Willett, Walter C., and Rudolph L. Leibel. "Dietary Fat Is Not a Major Determinant of Body Fat." *The American Journal of Medicine* 113, no. 9B (December 30, 2002): 47S–59S. https://doi.org/10.1016/s0002-9343(01)00992-5.

7. Dinicolantonio, James J., Sean C. Lucan, and James H. O'Keefe. "The Evidence for Saturated Fat and for Sugar Related to Coronary Heart Disease." *Progress in Cardiovascular Diseases* 58, no. 5 (2016): 464–72. https://doi.org/10.1016/j.pcad.2015.11.006.

8. Sumithran, P., L. A. Prendergast, E. Delbridge, K. Purcell, A. Shulkes, A. Kriketos, and J. Proietto. "Ketosis and Appetite-Mediating Nutrients and Hormones after Weight Loss." *European Journal of Clinical Nutrition* 67 (2013): 759–64. https://doi.org/10.1038/ejcn.2013.90.

9. Puchalska, Patrycja, and Peter A. Crawford. "Multi-Dimensional Roles of Ketone Bodies in Fuel Metabolism, Signaling, and Therapeutics." *Cell Metabolism* 25, no. 2 (February 7, 2017): 262–84. https://doi.org/10.1016/j.cmet.2016.12.022.

10. Teicholz, Nina. "Exit Trans Fats, Enter Something Worse?" Chapter. In *The Big Fat Surprise: Why Butter, Meat, and Cheese Belong in a Healthy Diet,* 275–81. New York, NY: Simon & Schuster Paperbacks, 2015. Kindle.

11. Schulte, Erica M., Nicole M. Avena, and Ashley N. Gearhardt. "Which Foods May Be Addictive? The Roles of Processing, Fat Content, and Glycemic Load." *PLoS ONE* 10, no. 2 (February 18, 2015). https://doi.org/10.1371/journal.pone.0117959.

Chapter 7

1. Suez, Jotham, Tal Korem, Gili Zilberman-Schapira, Eran Segal, and Eran Elinav. "Non-Caloric Artificial Sweeteners and the Microbiome: Findings and Challenges." *Gut Microbes* 6, no. 2 (2015): 149–55. https://doi.org/10.1080/19490976.2015.1017700.

2. Ruiz-Ojeda, Francisco Javier, Julio Plaza-Díaz, Maria Jose Sáez-Lara, and Angel Gil. "Effects of Sweeteners on the Gut Microbiota: A Review of Experimental Studies and Clinical Trials." *Advances in Nutrition* 10, no. suppl_1 (January 2019): S31–S48. https://doi.org/10.1093/advances/nmy037.

3. Dhillon, Jaapna, Janice Y. Lee, and Richard D. Mattes. "The Cephalic Phase Insulin Response to Nutritive and Low-Calorie Sweeteners in Solid and Beverage Form." *Physiology & Behavior* 181 (November 1, 2017): 100–09. https://doi.org/10.1016/j.physbeh.2017.09.009.

4. Just, Tino, Hans Wilhelm Pau, Ulrike Engel, and Thomas Hummel. "Cephalic Phase Insulin Release in Healthy Humans after Taste Stimulation?" *Appetite* 51, no. 3 (November 2008): 622–27. https://doi.org/10.1016/j.appet.2008.04.271.

5. Sinha, Rohit A., Benjamin L. Farah, Brijesh K. Singh, Monowarul M. Siddique, Ying Li, Yajun Wu, Olga R. Ilkayeva, et al. "Caffeine Stimulates Hepatic Lipid Metabolism by the Autophagy-Lysosomal Pathway in Mice." *Hepatology* 59, no. 4 (April 2014): 1366–80. https://doi.org/10.1002/hep.26667.

6. Pietrocola, Federico, Shoaib Ahmad Malik, Guillermo Mariño, Erika Vacchelli, Laura Senovilla, Kariman Chaba, Mireia Niso-Santano, Maria Chiara Maiuri, Frank Madeo, and Guido Kroemer. "Coffee Induces Autophagy in Vivo." *Cell Cycle* 13, no. 12 (March 2014): 1987–94. https://doi.org/10.4161/cc.28929.

7. Acheson, K. J., B. Zahorska-Markiewicz, P. Pittet, K. Anantharaman, and E. Jéquier. "Caffeine and Coffee: Their Influence on Metabolic Rate and Substrate Utilization in Normal Weight and Obese Individuals." *The American Journal of Clinical Nutrition* 33, no. 5 (May 1980): 989–97. https://doi.org/10.1093/ajcn/33.5.989.

8. Freedman, Neal D., Yikyung Park, Christian C. Abnet, Albert R. Hollenbeck, and Rashmi Sinha. "Association of Coffee Drinking with Total and Cause-Specific Mortality." *New England Journal of Medicine* 366, no. 20 (May 17, 2012): 1891–1904. https://doi.org/10.1056/nejmoa1112010.

9. Huxley, Rachel, Crystal Man Ying Lee, Federica Barzi, Leif Timmermeister, Sebastien Czernichow, Vlado Perkovic, Diederick E. Grobbee, David Batty, and Mark Woodward. "Coffee, Decaffeinated Coffee, and Tea Consumption in Relation to Incident Type 2 Diabetes Mellitus." *Archives of Internal Medicine* 169, no. 22 (December 14, 2009): 2053–63. https://doi.org/10.1001/archinternmed.2009.439.

10. Dulloo, A. G., C. A. Geissler, T. Horton, A. Collins, and D. S. Miller. "Normal Caffeine Consumption: Influence on Thermogenesis and Daily Energy Expenditure in Lean and Postobese Human Volunteers." *The American Journal of Clinical Nutrition* 49, no. 1 (January 1989): 44–50. https://doi.org/10.1093/ajcn/49.1.44.

11. Liu, Qing-Ping, Yan-Feng Wu, Hong-Yu Cheng, Tao Xia, Hong Ding, Hui Wang, Ze-Mu Wang, and Yun Xu. "Habitual Coffee Consumption and Risk of Cognitive Decline/Dementia: A Systematic Review and Meta-Analysis of Prospective Cohort Studies." *Nutrition* 32, no. 6 (June 2016): 628–36. https://doi.org/10.1016/j.nut.2015.11.015.

12. James, Jack E. "Critical Review of Dietary Caffeine and Blood Pressure: A Relationship That Should Be Taken More Seriously." *Psychosomatic Medicine* 66, no. 1 (2004): 63–71. https://doi.org/10.1097/10.psy.0000107884.78247.f9.

13. Mitrou, Panayota, Eleni Petsiou, Emilia Papakonstantinou, Eirini Maratou, Vaia Lambadiari, Panayiotis Dimitriadis, Filio Spanoudi, Sotirios A. Raptis, and George Dimitriadis. "Vinegar Consumption Increases Insulin-Stimulated Glucose Uptake by the Forearm Muscle in Humans with Type 2 Diabetes." *Journal of Diabetes Research* 2015 (May 6, 2015). https://doi.org/10.1155/2015/175204.

14. White, Andrea M., and Carol S. Johnston. "Vinegar Ingestion at Bedtime Moderates Waking Glucose Concentrations in Adults With Well-Controlled Type 2 Diabetes." *Diabetes Care* 30, no. 11 (November 2007): 2814–15. https://doi.org/10.2337/dc07-1062.

15. Vieira, Alexandra Ferreira, Rochelle Rocha Costa, Rodrigo Cauduro Oliveira Macedo, Leandro Coconcelli, and Luiz Fernando Martins Kruel. "Effects of Aerobic Exercise Performed in Fasted v. Fed State on Fat and Carbohydrate Metabolism in Adults: a Systematic Review and Meta-Analysis." *British Journal of Nutrition* 116, no. 7 (October 2016): 1153–64. https://doi.org/10.1017/s0007114516003160.

16. Proeyen, Karen Van, Karolina Szlufcik, Henri Nielens, Koen Pelgrim, Louise Deldicque, Matthijs Hesselink, Paul P. Van Veldhoven, and Peter Hespel. "Training in the Fasted State Improves Glucose Tolerance during Fat-Rich Diet." *The Journal of Physiology* 588, no. 21 (November 2010): 4289–302. https://doi.org/10.1113/jphysiol.2010.196493.

17. University of Bath. "Increase Health Benefits of Exercise by Working out before Breakfast." ScienceDaily, last modified October 18, 2019. https://www.sciencedaily.com/releases/2019/10/191018080619.htm.

18. Chaouachi, Anis, Aaron J. Coutts, Karim Chamari, Del P. Wong, Mustapha Chaouachi, Moktar Chtara, Rachida Roky, and Mohamed Amri. "Effect of Ramadan Intermittent Fasting on Aerobic and Anaerobic Performance and Perception of Fatigue in Male Elite Judo Athletes." *Journal of Strength and Conditioning Research* 23, no. 9 (December 2009): 2702–09. https://doi.org/10.1519/jsc.0b013e3181bc17fc.

19. Bock, K. De, W. Derave, B. O. Eijnde, M. K. Hesselink, E. Koninckx, A. J. Rose, P. Schrauwen, A. Bonen, E. A. Richter, and P. Hespel. "Effect of Training in the Fasted State on Metabolic Responses during Exercise with Carbohydrate Intake." *Journal of Applied Physiology* 104, no. 4 (April 2008): 1045–55. https://doi.org/10.1152/japplphysiol.01195.2007.

20. Zouhal, Hassane, Ayoub Saeidi, Amal Salhi, Huige Li, M. Faadiel Essop, Ismail Laher, Fatma Rhibi, Sadegh Amani-Shalamzari, and Abderraouf Ben Abderrahman. "Exercise Training and Fasting: Current Insights." *Open Access Journal of Sports Medicine* 11 (2020): 1–28. https://doi.org/10.2147/oajsm.s224919.

INDEX